PRESCRIPTION for INJURY

AF598813

The Politics of Pharmaceutical Manufacture, Regulation and Prescription

By

Colin Downes-Grainger

AMAD

Action Against Mind-Altering Drugs

Thanks to—
Ray Nimmo of benzo.org.uk, who has produced a unique benzodiazepine library online and has helped many victims over the years.

Charles Medawar of Social Audit who wrote the first illuminating text on the history of benzodiazepines and who has played a vital part in opening up the background of benzodiazepines and antidepressants.

The Beat the Benzos campaigning group and benzact.org.uk who bearded the Court of Screwed Medicine so persistently over the years, and the other selfless voluntary groups and individuals who soldiered on in the face of indifference.

Academics with independent and open minds, most notably Professor C.H. Ashton, Professor David Healy, Professor Malcolm Lader, Professor Andrew Herxheimer and Dr Aubrey Blumsohn.

Especial thanks to my wife Christine who provided 35 years of support and showed invaluable expertise in the formatting of the book.

Copyright © 2007 Colin Downes-Grainger
All rights reserved.

The moral right of the author has been asserted.

This edition published 2010 by Christine Downes-Grainger
Copyright ©

Printed and bound by http://www.fast-print.net/store.php
Peterborough PE2 6XD UK

Contents

Foreword

> Corporation, n. An ingenious device for obtaining profit without individual responsibility
> Ambrose Bierce 1842–1914, The Devil's Dictionary 1906

> "Let me give you the definition of ethics: it is good to maintain life and to further life. It is bad to damage and destroy life. And this ethic, profound and universal, has the significance of a religion. It is religion."
> Albert Schweitzer M.D; OM, 1875–1965, theologian, musician, philosopher, and physician

This book examines the politics of medical drugs and tells the story of how at least 17,000 people died and thousands more were permanently disabled because of the use of one class of drugs—the benzodiazepines. It highlights the story of thousands of state and doctor created victims who went through a drug induced hell when they took these prescribed and state-licensed drugs. These drugs cured nothing but caused much, and therefore arguments centred on risk/benefit did not and do not apply. Doctors were safeguarded against the reality of the harm they were causing by many factors, including the lack of time they spent with patients. They were also protected by an acquired and wrongheaded belief that no drug, as potentially harmful as patients said it was, would ever have been licensed without safeguards. The absence from manufacturer data sheets of the side-effect symptoms that patients were bringing into the surgery was a further guarantee of defence. The most important protection that prescribers have had, however, is the denial and smokescreen created by the Department of Health.

The history of benzodiazepines like Valium and Ativan is the story of how drug companies gave birth to the scandal through their influence with doctors, the policing of alternative views of the drugs, the controlling of government through ties with the regulatory bodies and advisers, and their use of power and money to ensure that legal actions became mired in procedure and ultimately failed, allowing the harm to continue unchecked.

Because of drug company activities, benzodiazepine prescribing and use became so widespread and of such long standing that denial of the realities and the employment of twisted logic and statistics, seemed to successive governments to be the logical course of action.

For denial to work, it became necessary for government to do several things, including not setting up dedicated withdrawal facilities, for to do that would be to admit that the drugs being prescribed by doctors were wreaking huge health and social damage on the British population. It was also necessary to ensure that the benzodiazepines were not rescheduled as dangerous drugs, for this would send a clear message out to the public and media, that an admission was being made that drugs which had been defended for so long and prescribed so widely, were infinitely damaging to health in the way they had and were being used.

They accepted that the medical profession policed itself as far as prescribing went, thus allowing a professional self protection mode to operate as a defence against patients, their representatives and campaigners. Related to this, they made sure that the system of patient complaints was difficult, where the first complaint had to be made to the offending doctor. The employers of doctors, known as Primary Care Trusts (PCTs), were the second port of call for complaint, but here, by allowing these Trusts to avoid responsibilities for checking on doctor prescribing, they made sure that PCTs had a motive for dismissing and avoiding patient complaints.

A series of cosmetic policies around the benzodiazepine scandal were undertaken. The Department of Health (DoH) employed an expert policy adviser on benzodiazepines, Dr Anna Higgitt, but because no apparent control of prescribing took place after her appointment, it seems likely this was more to do with informing the denial than with protecting future patients and holding out a helping hand to those who had been harmed historically. Part of the new approach was to create a stock reply to all those who corresponded with the Department. Any attempt at any time to engage with any individual at the DoH on the subject of benzodiazepine damage, even with new argument and evidence, meets with exactly the same response as that produced in the past. Summarised, this response has been: 'Yes we know there is a serious problem, and we take it very seriously...We are afraid that beyond the issuance of guidance and infrequent reminders, there is nothing we can do to prevent iatrogenic injury.'

When asked about help in withdrawal, Hazel Blears, before she moved on to greater glory in the Home Office and the Labour Party, had shamelessly maintained that help was available in drug misuse centres but it was not. Rosie Winterton, her successor, refined this message, perhaps having understood the view of campaigners that addicts created by doctors had no place in drug misuse treatment centres. Post Winterton, help was seemingly available in both primary and secondary settings—in GP surgeries, in psychiatric hospitals and through pharmacy advisers and specially employed nurses. If this had been true it would have been something, but lo and behold, in most areas of the country most of this provision did not exist. What kind of health system is it that deliberately misunderstands the 'problem', makes a pretence of action and asserts that psychiatry is an appropriate way to deal with drug-induced illness?

The phrase 'there is no evidence' is the most useful in the establishment lexicon. To the uninformed it means what it says—there is no evidence, the implication being that no evidence can be found. But what if the evidence was never looked for; what if evidence is hidden; what if the boundaries for acceptable evidence are circumscribed and narrow, what if evidence is deliberately not collated?

The harm done to patients over nearly half a century by benzodiazepine prescribing has been described as a scandal which has been covered up by government after government. It may be hard for some to believe that such a primary area of government provision as healthcare involves layers of mendacity, but the facts speak otherwise. The National Health Service is a political creation and its image is dear to both politicians and public. To acknowledge and make it known that the service does great harm to some, while benefiting others, is not something either government or doctors wish to dwell on. There are two other factors—the image of doctors and the protection of pharmaceutical companies.

Doctors are a scarce resource in the UK but their power to interpret and control events and information is far greater than their numbers might suggest. GPs are the foot soldiers of the NHS, its primary resource, and any suggestion that the majority have consistently acted without regard to patient safety, consigning thousands who were healthy to the scrapheap, is not something they would wish known. Ironically that fact is not something the public might want to hear either, particularly in this new age of consumer addiction to the idea of eternal good health through medicine.

Pharmaceutical companies are at the centre of the new health religion—no capitalist enterprise apart from perhaps the arms industry, has achieved such unaccountable power and influence with government. They have wrapped defences around their enterprise, of such depth and effectiveness that criticism of their activities—even from those who have been involved in their assault—is judged to be nothing more than a minority expression of a medical debate on the safety of medicines.

There are winners and losers in allopathic medicine and the providers of it would rather we did not dwell on the circumstances of the latter. In a glass cabinet at University College London, can be found the stuffed body of the 18th Century philosopher Jeremy Bentham, the man who created the notion of 'the greatest good for the greatest number'. That notion lives in the medical concept of risk/benefit with its recognisable undertones of ideas found in accountancy and economics, becoming 'the least harm for the greatest number'.

This may sound a fine and worthy philosophy, but when those who manufacture medicines have tailored their methods and goals towards the making of ever greater profit, when those who regulate the medicines are linked to the makers, when those who prescribe the medicines are educated by the makers and those who take the medicines remain uninformed of the risks they take—a new picture emerges. The philosophy of medicine then becomes 'the least admitted harm for the greatest number'.

The German pathologist Rudolf Virchow said in 1848 that politics was nothing more than medicine on a grand scale. He could equally have said had he lived now, that medicine is nothing more than politics on a grand scale. It is hard to know where one begins and the other ends, they appear to be interdependent.

This book is dedicated to those who have not benefited from medicine and its politics, but have become the losers. Many benzodiazepine victims have seamlessly gone on to become the victims of further prescribed drugs. These patients are people who found themselves on the wrong side of the risk/benefit scales, but then they were never aware that the scales were unbalanced and manufactured by vested interests. They believed, as do most still, in the benefits of medicine and the expert views of its providers.

Introduction

> "The scale of the [benzodiazepine] problem is so large...that it is beyond the grasp of many politicians and people in power to solve it. I think there's a paradox here, because you have this huge problem with a huge number of people involved, and yet we seem as a society to be incapable of acting on it. We can only cope with problems that are so big...we can't cope with this one."
> Phil Woolas MP, Local Government Minister,
> Croydon Conference, 2000

On October 1 1960, two doctors, Ingram and Timbury, of Southern General Hospital, Glasgow, wrote to the Lancet. They said:

> "A new tranquillising drug, (Librium), is now available commercially. It has been widely advertised in terms of its taming effect on wild animals and claims have been made that it is of special value in controlling phobic and obsessional symptoms in psychoneurosis although the published evidence for this is slight.
> Nine outpatients with phobic anxiety states and six with obsessional neuroses have been treated with this substance for three weeks. The dosage given was 10mg thrice daily for the first week and 25mg thrice daily thereafter. Only three of the nine phobic patients and one of the six obsessional neurotics felt any subjective improvement.
> Side-effects were seen in over half the patients. Two felt drowsy on the smaller dose, five on the larger. Two felt fatigued and apathetic, and dizziness and constipation were reported. One patient felt more energetic and two complained of severe irritability. After taking the drug for a week a schoolteacher struck his wife for the first time in the twenty years of their marriage. Of the fifteen patients, three had to stop work because of the side-effects and two others refused to continue taking the drug after two weeks.
> Although the number treated is small and the findings uncontrolled, the results are disappointing enough and the side-effects sufficiently troublesome to deserve attention.

> Other side-effects reported in trials in the United States have included dissociative reactions, hyperactivity, and ataxia.
> We feel justified in suggesting that the drug should be used with circumspection and scepticism until the results of controlled trials are available."

In the years following this report, prescriptions for Librium and its successors reached astronomical proportions, peaking in 1978 with nearly 31 million. Such has been the attention paid to those who were **not** hypnotised by the pharmaceutical claims of wonder and benefit.

Imagine these headlines:

'DOCTORS TURN WELL INTO SICK
WITH TRANQUILLISERS SHOCK!'

'DOCTORS KILL THOUSANDS
THOUSANDS MORE UNABLE TO WORK
FAMILIES IN DESPAIR!'

No one has ever seen these headlines, but they should have—this book presents the evidence that such headlines would have been more than justified.

Stories have appeared in the print media for many years—most in the local press, but none have examined the political backdrop to the occurrence and continuance of the injury to patients and their families. Instead the media has preferred to follow the human interest line, concentrating on the experiences of suffering of individuals. At this level they did provide a warning (for those who read them), but in the surgery, faced with a doctor telling them that it was all media hysteria, many who would have known better, unfortunately succumbed to this positive medical assurance. This added to the ever-growing number of casualties. The media coverage made no one aware that behind it all was an unexamined situation where the pharmaceutical industry controlled vital aspects of drugs regulation, political action and information to doctors.

The BBC and Independent broadcasters have explored the issue in programmes with titles such as 'The Tranquilliser Trap', or even 'Killer Pills', but these too did not reach the conclusions they might have reached. Again they concentrated largely on the personal story angle and levelled far too little criticism at the Department of Health, drug companies and the medical establishment. The BBC expressed astonishment that the DoH had no figures on addiction levels and that doctors routinely ignored the regulatory guidelines, issued in 1988, on safe prescribing. What they did not do was explore the reasons **why** guidelines were being ignored, or why it had taken nearly twenty-five years to issue them. The question of why the guidelines were issued has never been asked—what research evidence they were based on and when this evidence was produced. They did not express incredulity when government declared itself unable to control events in any direct way. They did not question the assurance that addiction withdrawal is not really a difficult problem, when in fact for many it is as much a horror story as it is with SSRI patients today, often taking years, with no assurance of complete recovery. One contributor expressed this aspect clearly in a response to 'The Tranquilliser Trap':

> "Why don't any of the programmes...on the subject of Benzodiazepines shown on the television tell the story of those/us that are left with the horrendous withdrawal effects for years after full withdrawal from these drugs?...Why doesn't the programme that you portray as supposedly for and to help the people of this country show the devastation caused by these drugs and not the pathetic description of addiction that was shown last night on your Panorama programme?"

No broadcast or print story has ever insisted that government explains how it reconciles what patients tell it about withdrawal horror with the fact that it has not seen fit to provide crucial support for those affected, and why it prefers to pretend that what exists is adequate and effective.

No examination has asked why tranquillisers are illegal drugs outside the surgery, or why they are Class C drugs, when less harmful drugs rank higher on the drug classification scale.

Programmes and print media, with the exception of a 2003 piece in the Observer, called 'Unhappy Anniversary', have never sought to discover what the standard of the science that led to the licensing of the drugs was, whether addiction potential was studied, or whether there had been long-term studies to determine the consequences of long-term prescribing.

Significantly, no one has ever explored the disparity between the experiences of tens of thousands of patients and what doctors believe about the drugs. Why, after nearly half a century, have no details of any controlled trials been released to the general public? Why will the Department of Health not fund clinical trials into the claims of damage of benzodiazepine long-term addicts and former addicts, affected as a result of taking the drugs?

The basic question of course is why medicine, which is associated in the public mind with healing, has, with the use of tranquillisers and hypnotics, inflicted such enormous harm to both the health and socio-economic lives of trusting patients. Medicine occupies one of the most crucial niches in society and yet experience over the years of the giant pharmaceutical companies has shown that medicine possesses a unique immunity to the consequences of its actions. Only the patient, it appears, is expected to bear the consequences of drugs, which the government licenses and its doctors prescribe.

Tranquilliser damage was not an accident. American based pharmaceutical companies, principally Wyeth and Roche, brought their marketing skills to bear on all aspects of licensing and doctor information. They controlled regulators through insider contacts, glossy pseudo-science and through the fact that many regulators owed their career positions and influence to their involvement with the industry. When the potential for damage became known through independent research and the observations of a minority of prescribers, they relied on their out-of-balance power in law, and the cowardice and self-interest of politicians who hid their heads in the sand. They relied too on the partiality of regulators, and the inadequacies of regulatory powers. Indeed, politicians, rather than improve the situation, made sure that the damage would continue, by ensuring that redress would be near impossible to secure through legal means. They restricted the ability of patients to take legal action against pharmaceutical companies and neglected to inform outdated legal assumptions about the nature of the damage.

Thalidomide damage ended only because the consequences were observable and undeniable. Psychotropic drug damage is a different kettle of fish. By maintaining the illusion that tranquillisers are drugs associated only with clinical anxiety and minimising recognition of the damage, government and regulators have been able to assert that withdrawal and problems during prescription have been the unfortunate downside of a necessary medication. They and the manufacturers have had no incentive to explore the claims of patients about the reality of a much greater damage than the limited range of symptoms acknowledged.

Tranquillisers were marketed as safe and non-addictive. When it became impossible to deny any longer that they were not, government and regulators allowed manufacturers to drip feed supposedly newly found possible side-effects, over years and decades. No government instructed its regulators to examine the science in detail, looking for drug company evasion. No government has ever seen the necessity to provide research funding to examine patient claims. No government has ever insisted that manufacturers held any kind of responsibility. No government has ever veered from the line that doctors always had the best interests of patients at heart, and that by and large they prescribed appropriately—this even while doctors were rejecting safety guidelines and no rigorous science demonstrated long-term safety.

It does not matter whether you live in America, Canada, New Zealand, Australia or any other point of the compass, the picture of drugs' regulation owing its first duty to manufacturers as its clients, remains the same. This is because politicians have vested interests in the continuing health of the pharmaceutical industry, which was described by Dr Robert Hare, adviser to the FBI on psychopaths, as having all the characteristics of the psychopath. Governments could formulate a system of regulation that works but they do not. In the UK, how regulation operates is a subject that rivals the processes of MI6 or the CIA. Secrecy is a very useful barrier against change.

It is known from government figures (not the Department of Health), that tranquillisers have killed thousands of people, not as many as barbiturates perhaps, but more than enough.

Tranquillisers have devastated an untold number of lives—they have destroyed patients, marriages and families. They are often amazingly difficult to withdraw from completely, and the hidden cost to the NHS and to society is incalculable. The addiction has been made far worse by the ignorance and denial of doctors, based not on scientific evidence, merely the absence of regulatory action and the assurances of pharmaceutical companies.

Many tranquilliser addicts have been too frightened to relate growing mental problems to their GPs for fear of being consigned to psychiatric hospitals, too frightened to reduce their intake because they have known that even reduced functioning required the maintenance of prescriptions, too frightened to question the effect of the pills for the same reason.

Cocktails of drugs have been prescribed to counteract the unrecognised effects of benzodiazepines—mistakenly diagnosed and treated as new illnesses, increasing the damage done through drugs.

Professionalism and dedication to patient protection does not figure largely in official circles it seems. Not only has government allowed the benzodiazepine situation to continue over almost half a century but it has demonstrated a complete unwillingness to find out the true extent of the problem which it says it recognises and takes seriously. These are questions (among many) it could ask and seek answers to, but does not:

- Benzodiazepine reactions mimic other illnesses so at any one time, how many hospital admissions involve patients taking these drugs?
- Why are Patient Information Leaflets so uninformative and anodyne?
- How many children being given Ritalin by doctors are the children of mothers who took benzodiazepines?
- How many disability benefit and incapacity claimants are on long-term prescribed tranquillisers and hypnotics?
- Recovered alcoholics and heroin addicts, who have also taken benzodiazepines, routinely declare that tranquilliser withdrawal is far worse than any other type of drug withdrawal. Why is it that the proponents of the benzodiazepine protocol find it easy to maintain its benefit?

- When it is well known that benzodiazepines can precipitate suicide, aggression and are a serious cause of a variety of accidents, why is it not compulsory to test for their presence in all such cases?
- Why do patients and campaigners continue to insist that withdrawal assistance does not exist?
- Why do doctors banish 'difficult' tranquilliser patients from their surgeries?
- Why does the UK legal system effectively prevent a doctor or drug company being sued for the damage they have inflicted on patients?
- Why does drug regulation repeatedly allow medical damage?

It is impossible for anyone to empathise with all the scandals they are faced with in society, still less act on them. Instead we may sympathise but then leave it to those involved, and those whose duty it is to make changes and protect the innocent. It is important, however, to understand that a system which has allowed such enormous damage is a system with a history. It has always allowed drug damage and washed its hands afterwards. It has not, even now, changed in its essentials, and without protest and the signalling of disapproval, it will never change. You may not have been personally involved in the tranquilliser tragedy or in the ongoing antidepressant situation, but if in the future you receive a prescription, you would like to know that the drug really is as safe as it could possibly be made. Wouldn't you?

The Problem Explained

"There's no scientific evidence to indicate that one particular tranquilliser is worse than another. To act just against one would be wrong because there is a problem with the whole group."
Professor Michael Rawlins, member of the Committee on the Safety of Medicines and Chair of its Subcommittee on Safety, Efficacy and Adverse Reactions, Brass Tacks, BBC2, October 20 **1987**

"Millions of people are being turned into life long addicts by doctors who continue to ignore prescribing guidelines. Because those affected don't have to steal to fund their habit, but instead get the drugs from the health service, their plight goes largely unnoticed by society. But the cost of family breakdowns and individual impairment is immense."
Chris Davies MEP, **2004**

"There is a lack of support and rehabilitation services available for people still addicted to benzodiazepine drugs, many of whom were first prescribed them in the 1970s or 1980s. Not a single NHS benzodiazepine rehabilitation clinic exists in the UK today."
House of Commons Health Committee, **2005**

"The issue of benzodiazepine addiction is a serious one and I have discussed it with my colleagues. There are a large number of pressing issues affecting the health service at this time. Unfortunately it is not possible for us to undertake an inquiry along the lines you suggest."
Kevin Barron MP, Chairman, House of Commons Health Committee, 24 April **2007**

As far as responsibility for health damage through drug prescribing is concerned, the finger constantly points in someone else's direction. But if there is no responsibility taken in any quadrant, who in fact owns responsibility? In 1999, Charles Medawar of Social Audit told 'Face the Facts', on BBC Radio 4:

> "Given that many benzodiazepine users tend to be elderly and their life expectation is not all that high, there is no incentive to reduce costs by reducing the amount of dependence. I've no doubt that if benzodiazepine dependence were a very expensive social problem solutions would and could be found."

But was he only partly right? Are benzodiazepine drugs in fact a **very** expensive social problem? There are somewhere around 160,000 illicit benzodiazepine drug users—90% of all illicit users also ingest or inject benzodiazepines. Over-prescribing has led to a burgeoning black market in supply and demand.

According to the Department of Health, it is Primary Care Trusts that are responsible for the provision of services, depending on local needs—but these services do not exist—though there are some services for illicit users. Government provides no dedicated finance for local services, probably for political reasons, and in the present economic climate, with a cash-strapped NHS cutting mental health services around the country, it is impossible to believe that PCTs would prioritise assistance.

There is an establishment promoted myth that people suffer only from 'anxiety' during withdrawal. Belief in this myth is understandable since it has been disseminated by UK politicians and drug regulators and largely accepted by the media. Since 1960, the UK medical profession through its profligate prescribing has routinely turned hundreds of thousands of healthy people into addicts, many with brain damage, and then turned its back on the situation it created. There are currently around one million addicted patients and uncounted thousands disabled by withdrawal.

Addicted patients, because of the sedative nature of tranquillisers, are normally quiescent individuals. Withdrawing ones are often extremely difficult, particularly in the view of those who addicted them. Over the half century of benzodiazepine prescribing, it has been the experience of patients involved that it was all too easy for the medical profession to ignore and dismiss patients who reported symptoms and sought help and explanations. Disability benefits for people who were once well, before they came into contact with prescribers are not normally available, since it is a medical profession in denial that decides whether the disability exists. Seriously ill patients are cast aside, doctors finding it easy to see them as suffering from a 'mental problem'.

The current theory proposed by Professor Heather Ashton regarding protracted withdrawal symptoms is that benzodiazepines destroy and deplete GABA/Benzodiazepine receptors. There are people who start life with high concentrations, average concentrations and low concentrations. Those with low concentrations are hit hardest and are the group who will most sustain permanent damage from tranquillisers. The former President

of the Royal College of Psychiatrists admitted in the British Medical Journal in 2003, that patients had reported over 200 different adverse reactions to the drugs. This list of withdrawal effects was written by Professor Jeffrey Richards, at the University of Ballarat in Australia.
http://www.med.monash.edu.au/non-cms/mentalhealth/benzos/

Common Withdrawal Symptoms
Abdominal pains and cramps
Agoraphobia
Anxiety
Breathing Difficulties
Blurred Vision
Changes in Perception
Depression
Distended Abdomen
Dizziness
Extreme Lethargy
Irritability
Lack of concentration
Lack of coordination
Loss of balance
Loss of memory
Muscular aches and pains
Nausea
Nightmares
Rapid mood changes (crying one minute and then laughing)
Fears (uncharacteristic)
Restlessness
Feelings of unreality
Severe headaches
Flu-like symptoms
Shaking
Heavy limbs
Seeing spots
Heart palpitations
Sore eyes
Hypersensitivity to light
Sweating
Indigestion
Tightness in chest
Insomnia
Tightness in the head (feeling a band around the head)

Less Common Withdrawal Symptoms
Aching jaw
Numbness in any body part
Craving for sweet food
Outbursts of rage and aggression
Constipation
Diarrhoea
Paranoia
Depersonalisation (a feeling of not knowing who you are)
Painful scalp
Persistent, unpleasant memories
Pins and needles
Difficulty swallowing
Rapid body changes in temperature
Feelings of the ground moving
Sexual problems
Hallucinations (auditory and visual)
Skin problems
Hyperactivity
Hypersensitivity to sound
Speech difficulties
Sore mouth and tongue
Suicidal thoughts
Incontinence or frequency or urgency
Increased saliva

Rare Withdrawal Symptoms
Blackouts
Bleeding from the nose
Burning along the spine
Craving for pills
Discharge from the breasts
Falling hair
Haemorrhoids
Hypersensitivity to touch
Rectal bleeding
Sinus pain
Seizures
Sensitive or painful teeth

The medical profession has escaped responsibility, because it has never been controlled or held responsible by government and because of the public myth that doctors know what they are doing when they prescribe tranquillisers and other psychotropic medications. Government has in fact turned the world upside down and asserted—without evidence—that treatment has been readily available within the NHS and that doctors have acted responsibly. The profession has in addition been able to shelter under the umbrella of benzodiazepine manufacturers who have controlled awareness of what these drugs do, and regulators whose equations for the calculation of risk/benefit have no validity in the context of how these drugs have been prescribed.

It is quite clear from the long history of benzodiazepine damage to people's lives, that health protection is a case of smoke and mirrors. The mirrors reflect an absence of injury and this is trumpeted as large-scale benefit, but beyond the smoke is the area of health devastation. This area, though beyond the picture captured by the mirrors, is the experience of many. Those outside the experience of that devastation would never know it exists. It is in the interests, it seems, of no manufacturer, healthcare provider, prescriber or drugs regulator to reflect it. The Health Committee obviously does not see it as an area of responsibility and would seem to have no idea of what is meant by the term 'serious problem' as it applies to tranquillisers.

The 2004–5 inquiry into the Influence of the Pharmaceutical Industry by the Health Committee, made many useful recommendations on that issue but it should be noted that government rejected the key findings. The 'problem' of benzodiazepines occupied very little space in the report. Campaigners, including one minister, had failed to convince the committee that it was high time the issue was examined in detail. The response of the government was that it would be wrong to concentrate on one drug, ignoring the fact that campaigners had never asked for that—they had said that an examination of tranquillisers would provide a definitive picture of how drug companies sold their safety message and successfully controlled regulators and prescribers.

Attempts to penetrate the smoke and gain recognition are limited by many factors, not least of which is that responsibility for health safety is so widely spread. Those charged with the assessment of damage inflicted by drugs are the ones who license the drugs. In the UK it is the Medicines and Healthcare products Regulatory Agency (MHRA). There is, right from the start, an inherent conflict in these two roles and the only possible political defence uses references to the nobility of science and the scientists working within the MHRA. It seems not to matter how much evidence there is that the direction and use of pharmaceutical science is often more ignoble than noble, and that the MHRA is an amateur, self-serving organisation, staffed by people whose careers rose on the back of that science. The message of scientific endeavour for the benefit and safety of all must be maintained. The NHS is a political construct and is defended by politicians from any serious attempt to explore what it commonly does to patients through the blind prescribing of drugs.

But rather than a situation where an efficient, impartial group of scientifically trained people closely examine honest and rigorous evidence provided by drug manufacturers before they license a medicine—what happens is the opposite. The scientific evidence produced for the licensing of benzodiazepines was far from rigorous but since these drugs have been in use for nearly 50 years now, it might therefore seem that the fact that they have remained on pharmacy shelves, must mean that they are safe. This is far from true—they are still there because regulators have failed to act in any way effectively, drug companies have used their power to control the message, prescribers have been allowed by government to use clinical judgement in the face of independent scientific evidence, and politicians have seen the political consequence if any admission was ever made about their true nature. **The nub of the problem is that tens of thousands of people who were not sick, became sick through the prescription of medicines** which the manufacturers said were not addictive and were safe. SSRIs follow the same course today.

Many people have been taking these drugs for decades and have not only lost their health but also their economic and social well-being as a result. The nature of the drugs is such that after long-term prescription, many never recover major aspects of health or regain security and a place in society if they do withdraw. People were turned into addicts by drugs which are illegal outside the doctor's surgery, and many of them have effectively lost their whole lives. No doctor or representative group in the UK has ever held up their hands and said sorry, partly perhaps because government and its regulators have allowed them to go on believing that what they did was medically acceptable and the damage caused was not all that significant in the scale of things. The sad truth though, is that while the past has been glossed over and no one has responsibility for it, non-recognition of that past has allowed contemporary damage, through over-prescription, to continue.

The Victims

The following experiences are only a sample of personal experiences of benzodiazepines, and they are only the tip of the iceberg—a representation of what happens to individuals when prescribers are ignorant, regulators are compromised and government sees the protection of an industry which provides jobs and large-scale revenue as being more important than health protection.

The first are from 'The Tranquilliser Trap', a BBC programme broadcast on Sunday 13 May 2001:

> "I was prescribed Lorazepam at 16. I am now aged 44 and have been off tranquillisers for two years, after a GP

suggested that I had perhaps been on them too long! After suffering most of my life with Agoraphobia and Panic Attacks, I cannot believe that this drug is still manufactured. It is high time the drug companies were held accountable and something positive was done. How many people have to lose their quality of life and battle so hard, with little help to regain it, before someone says stop."

"I have been on this medication for 34 years, yes 34 years, and all because I had a small concern in 1967. All doctors told me was to keep taking the meds. One year ago I started to find out that I didn't need it. BUT to get off it is a serious job, people need help and advice. I nearly died of going into convulsions as I didn't know enough about how to withdraw. I'm still in a very serious condition called derealization, the doctor said it was like stopping smoking! I nearly killed myself."

"My doctor prescribed Librium continuously for 10 years in the 70–80s after a minor bout of anxiety. My memory is permanently impaired over that period."

"I was on those drugs for 10 years and I don't remember any of it. When I finally got off, it was like waking up. What happened to me was horrendous and it has affected my whole family. I'm still living with the effects."
Barry Haslam, Benzodiazepine Campaigner and Consultant

"I have been on Valium for 37 years and still no help. Doctors don't care for your health."

"I have been taking Nitrazepam for 20 years, I can't stop taking them. When I was given them by a hospital doctor I was told that they were to relax me so that I could sleep. I was not told anything about them being addictive. Obviously I have found out that they are highly addictive. If I do not take them my whole body shakes to such an extent that I cannot hold a cup of tea in my hand. I also get terrifying dreams, there is much more that I can tell you about them."

"If the government knows these drugs to be harmful why are they allowing them to be dispensed? Why have they not implemented resources to help patients come off the drugs. It takes more than a guideline...the problem will not go away...Indeed it will not 'die' off which is one method some

GPs are using to reduce their prescriptions, i.e. they are waiting for those patients who have been addicted for 20+ years to die because it is easier to give a 2 minute prescription rather than seeing a demanding patient for 20 minutes a visit every day until they get what they demand."

"My uncle was prescribed Ativan over 25 years ago. The doctor then prescribed practically every other drug that was mentioned on your fantastic insight in to this brushed under the carpet crime. He is agoraphobic, intense mood swings and all the symptoms the programme mentioned."

"I was left unmonitored on benzos for 17 years. Withdrawal was a nightmare—hallucinations & mania. I am appalled that the drug companies are not taken to task and forced to pay compensation. All medical experts now agree that they are addictive. No person, regardless of their initial mental health problems deserves the horror of benzodiazepine withdrawal."

"I believe I am one of the longest addicts of Lorazepam, I started taking them in 1974 following a car accident and finished taking them in 2000 (26 years). I was 18 when I was first prescribed them and the effect upon my life has been devastating, like others I thought I was going out of my mind, a fact my doctor was only too willing to agree with...I am forty five and I can't remember what it was like when I was 18, I can't remember a time when my life was not governed by fear. I may function in society, but that does not mean I can lead a normal life. However I find that the medical profession believes that now I no longer take these drugs that I am back to full fitness...I was offered no support from anywhere and yet if I was a Heroin addict, I would have had masses of help and support."

"It is rare to find any useful help out there from the same doctors that prescribed these things to millions of people over the years, including me. I have been working at getting off these for two years off and on and it is the hardest thing I have ever done."

"All that was missing was a more complete presentation of the dreadful after effects of withdrawal from dependency on prescription drugs such as diazepam. I was fed diazepam and a cocktail of other pills for thirty years and five years ago voluntarily stopped following advice in an article reprinted from an American medical journal. Five years on I have chronic pains in my legs which apparently defy diagnosis by UK GPs but is documented in the USA. In my opinion far too little work has been done in this area and it will be difficult to get people to withdraw unless they know that support is in place to cope with the after effects."

> "Many people in their 30s, 40s and 50s have now worked out that prescribed chemicals killed their parents and/or grandparents! The hidden cost to the world and its peoples in physical, mental, emotional and financial terms is inestimable!"

These experiences were recounted on 'Face the Facts', BBC Radio 4, March 16 1999:

> "I went to my doctor's and said: "Do they make you lose your memory?" And he said 'No.' My memory went down and down. I can't remember what I did yesterday and I don't think about tomorrow. There's no tomorrow—all there is, is now..."

> "I used to be a dancer and I got medals for dancing but I couldn't go back to dancing again and I just feel that I couldn't mix...I will never be the same person I was because I just feel I've been damaged."

> "It was one Saturday—my dad phoned me up and said: "You'll have to come to the hospital with your mum, she's had a fall." I made an excuse saying: "I'm going out but I'll give you a ring back to see how she is." Basically I just couldn't go out of the house. My son who was 21 at the time had to do the shopping for me. I couldn't even go to the corner shop."

> "She's gone from a very bright, athletic girl—a very intelligent, attractive girl, into almost a recluse and she looks ill all the time and she says she feels ill all the time. She doesn't go out, she doesn't do anything, she has no future, she has no career prospects, she has no life."

> "There are people out there...who are hooked, unknowingly, unwillingly, and they feel that society has 'chucked them overboard'. They feel they no longer belong anywhere. They feel they've lost such a lot, that they can no longer regard themselves as fully human."

> "You can say it in one really—I feel as if my own self—at some stage—was removed. I gradually went missing. My personality gradually went missing."

This was related by Ray Nimmo the founder of www.benzo.org.uk on the BBC Radio 4 programme, 'You and Yours', July 16 2002, 'Benzodiazepine Guidelines routinely ignored'.

> "I was just left on repeat prescriptions of these drugs. I was told that I was the problem—that I needed to stay on these drugs. I just became suicidally depressed, so anxious, agoraphobic, lethargic. I just didn't want to go out of the house. I didn't want to answer the door or the telephone. I was just like a zombie—living in this twilight world of paranoia and fear. It was dreadful...By March 1986 I just had to give up work. I couldn't cope with life let alone a career or a job of any kind. My family were just completely at a loss. My wife managed one day at a time—trying to look after me, managing all the household, doing all the shopping, looking after our young son. My son is 20 next month. I really don't even remember him for all those years. It's as if my whole memory is blotted out. It's as if all those 14 years happened to someone else..."

These are a selection of experiences recorded in print media over the years:

> "In the past forty years I haven't had a life...No one can say they've seen me go up the street on my own, or take my children out on my own, or go on a bus. When my daughter was at primary school, her teacher told her she couldn't understand why I never came to parents' evenings. If my mum hadn't been there to look after them, they would probably have been taken into care."
> Unhappy Anniversary of Valium,
> Observer, February 2 2003

> "She finds it difficult to concentrate and is crippled by a devastating fatigue that cuts short her activities and blights her life. The fall-out from weaning herself off the drugs has affected her husband Bob, 53, and other members of her family. "We have all suffered. I feel so sorry for Bob—I am surprised he has stuck with me," she said. She started off taking Valium and ended up being prescribed a whole cocktail of different drugs to combat the many side-effects. And when

she came off them, Val's problems just seemed to escalate. "There have been times when I have wished I could die. The pain has been so bad and I just don't seem to get any better. "Nobody can tell me why this has happened to me and worse still they can't tell me if it will ever end," she said."
'I wanted to die',
Southampton Daily Echo, April 18 2006

"After 30 years of tranquillisers mixed with a variety of antidepressants, the mother-of-six says the drugs have left her physically and mentally handicapped. Over the years Mrs Dixon's health has deteriorated and she has suffered a host of problems including panic attacks, muscle weakness, mood swings, bowel problems, nausea and severe pelvic pain. Her condition has left her unable to leave her home for the past 10 years and watch her children and 20 grandchildren growing up..."
'Grandma's tablet warning',
Newcastle Evening Chronicle, May 27 2004

"One Barnet woman, who wanted to remain anonymous, says she was left housebound after being addicted to benzodiazepines for more than 20 years. She was originally prescribed the drugs for a stomach upset, but now suffers thyroid problem, asthma, ME and leg pain so severe she can hardly walk—all of which she attributes to the drugs."
Tranquilliser addiction is 'damaging our health',
Hendon and Finchley Times, August 21 2003

"Jennifer describes her life as a living nightmare—a hellish version of reality that was brought on after withdrawing from 31 years of daily Valium use. She describes herself as a shadow of the woman she was before she started to come off the common tranquilliser more than two-and-a-half-years ago. "This isn't a life—I have no life of my own," she said. "I live my life like a hermit. I used to travel all over the world with my job. Now I can only just make it down the road to Abergavenny. Everything I enjoy in life I can't do anymore because of the depression. I have panic attacks if I'm left alone...It seems the only way out of this is death. I feel so hopeless.""
'Tranquilliser Hell still haunts patient after 31-year addiction',
The Western Mail, March 17 2003

"I started off on Valium in 1973 when I was 18." he says. "I had gone to the GP because I felt a bit shy and introverted. I was not a very outgoing fellow and there was some personal stuff in my childhood. I had anxiety, tension and stress. The doctor gave me Valium. I took it and felt that it was great. I felt very attached to it." So attached, that it was to dominate the next 14 years of his life. "For all that time, I was living in a haze. I lost my job and did not care. Once I had it I could float around. I stopped for a very short time and felt that the world was a frightening place...I did not realise that this was worse than a heroin addiction. It's very secretive as well. It's like putting on a mask. Behind it all you are a shell, dying inside."
Sunday Tribune, Ireland, March 2 2003

"The children spent their early years in and out of nurseries because I couldn't cope, and I missed out on so much of their childhood. They all deserve so much more, but I felt powerless to change. I vaguely remembered what I used to be like and wished I could get back to being my old self, but I couldn't stop taking the pills and I was scared I'd feel worse without them. Whenever I tried to come off them, I turned into a physical as well as an emotional wreck. I'd shake and sweat would pour off me. My body couldn't cope—I was addicted. Roy was desperate to help but my doctors couldn't offer any alternatives to the repeat prescriptions."
'I had to be drugged up to the eyeballs to function',
Best Magazine, February 20 2001

"Michael, 56, was first prescribed the tranquilliser Ativan, a benzodiazepine used to treat anxiety and insomnia, in 1977...He estimates he has 69 side-effects, including extreme sensitivity to light, sound and temperature, chronic bowel and intestinal problems, muscle aches, vertigo and insomnia. He can barely walk and hasn't left his home since August. The pain in his legs is so intense, that he can't bear anything to touch them."
Man's life 'blighted by pills',
York Evening Press, October 30 2000

"Ann Tallentyre was first prescribed benzodiazepines 32 years ago—and has been taking them ever since. 'I do not live, I exist,' she says. 'I can't go out because I have agoraphobia. I am totally dependent on others—my daughter has to do the shopping.'"

'Benzodiazepines can ruin lives', More addictive than heroin yet prescribed to one in four adults.
Sunday Express Magazine 1999

"Mr Morris was first given a tranquilliser at Royal Oldham Hospital after suffering a panic attack when his father died. His then GP continued the prescription for nearly six years. Mr Morris has since had 70 electrocardiograms for chest pains. He says: "I can't sleep, I am constantly sweating. I can't go out. I can't associate with people properly...The Royal Oldham would not comment on Mr Morris' case but said **the CSM guidelines were for advice only. Doctors were free to make clinical decisions."**
'Valium Father to sue',
Mail on Sunday, June 22 1997

"The practice of "switching the patients out with the lights" is causing increasing concern among medical and charitable organisations, according to the report by the Royal College of Physicians. More than 90 per cent of residents of the homes are prescribed drugs, and nearly half are taking major tranquillisers and other sedatives..."I fear that in some homes these drugs are being used like a chemical ball and chain to keep patients quiet. These are very frail physically and mentally ill people and virtually the entire lot are on medication, with a large proportion on sedatives. It is a growing cause for concern."
[Dr Michael Denham, Consultant Geriatrician at Northwick Park Hospital and chairman of the working party that produced the report]"
'Sedative cocktails fed to the elderly',
The Independent, May 7 1997

"Gwen Howard claims that tranquillisers have completely ruined her life. 'I was prescribed them for 17 years' says Gwen, a pensioner from Nottingham, who has started a support group for fellow sufferers. 'It changed my personality, ruined my life and destroyed my marriage. I was so ill I had to stop working 10 years ago, when I was only 54.'"
'I'm not asking for charity—just justice!'
Best Magazine, March 21 1995

"I had a successful teaching job once and my wife could have had a successful teaching career. Now at 60 and 58

respectively, after a 35 year experience of benzodiazepines, the best we can look forward to is a fundamentally insecure and impoverished old age, after a fundamentally insecure and impoverished previous three decades."
The Author, benzodiazepine victim and founder of AMAD, Action Against Mind-Altering Drugs

In the face of the evidence and decades of pleas from patients, the Department of Health has consistently failed to recognise the picture being described. Two statements have been churned out ad nauseam—we take the problem seriously, and our priority is to prevent addiction occurring. I suggest that to those outside politics, these statements have never addressed anything, and have in fact been nothing less than an affront to normal intelligence and an uncaring nonsense. They do not take the 'Problem Seriously'.

Primum non nocere is the Latin phrase that means "First, do no harm." The phrase is sometimes recorded as primum nil nocere. It is one of the principal precepts all medical students are taught in medical school. It is a reminder to a doctor that he or she must consider the possible harm that any intervention might do. It is most often mentioned when debating use of an intervention with an obvious chance of harm but a less certain chance of benefit.

From the Committee on the Review of Medicines quoted in The British Medical Journal, 29 March, **1980**:

> "The committee further noted that there was little convincing evidence that benzodiazepines were efficacious in the treatment of anxiety after four months' continuous treatment. It considered that an appropriate warning regarding long-term efficacy be included in the recommendations, particularly in view of the high proportion of patients receiving repeated prescriptions for extended periods of time.
> It further suggested that patients receiving benzodiazepine therapy be carefully selected and monitored and that prescriptions be limited to short-term use."

From the Committee on Safety of Medicines UK Government Bulletin to Prescribers, January **1988**:

> CURRENT PROBLEMS 1988; Number 21: 1–2
> BENZODIAZEPINES, DEPENDENCE AND WITHDRAWAL SYMPTOMS

There has been concern for many years regarding benzodiazepine dependence. (Br.Med.J.1980:280,910–912) Such dependence is becoming increasingly worrying. Withdrawal symptoms include anxiety, tremor, confusion, insomnia, perceptual disorders, fits, depression, gastrointestinal and other somatic symptoms. These may sometimes be difficult to distinguish from the symptoms of the original illness.

It is important to note that withdrawal symptoms can occur with benzodiazepines following therapeutic doses given for SHORT periods of time.

Withdrawal effects usually appear shortly after stopping a benzodiazepine with a short half life, or up to several days after stopping one with a long half life. Symptoms may continue for weeks or months.

No epidemiological evidence is available to suggest that one benzodiazepine is more responsible for the development of dependency or withdrawal symptoms than another.

The Committee on Safety of Medicines recommends that the use of benzodiazepines should be limited in the following way:

USES

As Anxiolytics

Benzodiazepines are indicated for the short-term relief (two to four weeks only) of anxiety that is severe, disabling or subjecting the individual to unacceptable distress, occurring alone or in association with insomnia or short-term psychosomatic, organic or psychotic illness. The use of benzodiazepines to treat short-term 'mild' anxiety is inappropriate and unsuitable.

As Hypnotics

Benzodiazepines should be used to treat insomnia only when it is severe, disabling, or subjecting the individual to extreme distress.

DOSE

The lowest dose which can control the symptoms should be used. It should not be continued beyond four weeks.

PRECAUTIONS

1. Benzodiazepines should not be used alone to treat depression or anxiety associated with depression. Suicide may be precipitated in such patients.
2. They should not be used for phobic or obsessional states.

> 3. They should not be used for the treatment of chronic psychosis.
> 4. In cases of loss or bereavement, psychological adjustment may be inhibited by benzodiazepines.
> Disinhibiting effects may be manifested in various ways. Suicide may be precipitated in patients who are depressed, and aggressive behaviour towards self and others may be precipitated. Extreme caution should therefore be used in prescribing benzodiazepines in patients with personality disorders.

It seems as though NHS doctors should have prescribed themselves reading glasses, they kept on prescribing.

> "Increasing numbers of people have been turned into drug addicts through legal prescriptions which perhaps suits the politicians and multi-national bureaucrats as well as the drug companies for it ensures an uncomplaining and docile community which is easy to administer, manage and manipulate...tranquillisers are more addictive than heroin."
> Dr Vernon Coleman, 'Life without Tranquillisers', 1985

> "The benzodiazepines are probably the most addictive drugs ever created and the vast army of enthusiastic doctors who prescribed these drugs by the tonne have created the world's largest drug addiction problem.
> Dr Vernon Coleman, 'The Drugs Myth', 1992

> "The British State is just drugging people into submission because they are less of a nuisance that way."
> Mathew Parris, journalist and former MP, 'For the Benefit of Mr Parris Revisited', ITV, 29 January 2004

Professor Malcolm Lader's accurate comments have charted a chunk of the history of benzodiazepine prescribing. Psychophamacologist Malcolm Lader was a member of the Committee on the Review of Medicines from 1978–1989:

> 1978: He described benzodiazepines as the opium of the masses.
> 1981: He said there was an epidemic in the making.

Prescribing doctors, as he observed, had enthusiastically taken up the 'use for everything' message coming from the manufacturers and the result was a huge edifice of state-countenanced addiction.

> 1982: He said he had evidence of shrunken brains from scans of long-term users.
> 1988: He said benzodiazepine addiction was the biggest medically-induced problem of the late 20th Century.

Lader was emphasising the crucial role played by medicine and its prescribers in creating not only an addiction problem which should never have existed, but also one instance of its terrible potential impact on physical health.

> 1991: He said no real attempt was being made to help addicts come off. Government should set aside funds.

He had now homed in on the fact that government had shown no real concern for what it had allowed to happen. At the very least, in the aftermath of what had gone on before, it should have provided help for the victims of the licensed drugs, but had not thought fit to do so. It has not found it possible to do so since.

In 1980 the Committee on the Review of Medicines (CRM) had said:

> **"...patients receiving benzodiazepine therapy be carefully selected and monitored and [that] prescriptions [should] be limited to short-term use."**

These are the prescription figures for the years **after** this statement was made. All figures are in Millions.

Benzodiazepines 1980–1988 in UK:

1980	29.1
1981	29.5
1982	29.7
1983	28.7
1984	28.0
1985	25.7
1986	25.3
1987	25.5
1988	23.2

In 1988 the CRM's successor, the Committee on Safety of Medicines (CSM) had said that tranquilliser dependence was increasingly worrying. But this was the prescription level **one year after** the Guidance:

1989 22.1

Twelve years after the CRM expert opinion, and **four years after** the Guidance issued by the CSM this was the prescription level:

1992 15.8

Fifteen years after the CRM expert opinion, and **seven years after** 1988, the level was still far too high:

1995 14.027

Twenty two years after the CRM expert opinion, and **fourteen years after** the CSM Guidance for doctors, Department of Health data showed that 30% of these prescriptions failed to adhere to it.

2002 12.7

Twenty five years after the CRM expert opinion, and **seventeen years after** the guidance from the CSM, the figures were still at a completely unsafe level:

2005 11.252

Government watched this happen and showed no real concern.

Benzodiazepine-related deaths

Professor Ashton commented in a January 2005 letter to MP Phil Woolas:

> "Official Home Office data shows 1800 benzodiazepine-related deaths during a six year period between 1990 and 1996, i.e. 300 deaths/year.
> Extrapolation of this data to the period 1964–2004 would suggest a figure of 12,000 such deaths.
> This figure is likely to be of the right order, considering that prescription numbers for Benzodiazepines were extremely high in the period 1970–1985 (reaching over 31 million/yr in the UK in 1978 compared with about 17 million at present)

> and, considering that Benzodiazepines are taken in over 40% of all self-poisonings and by over 50% of all polydrug abusers. Adding the observation that benzodiazepines cause 110 road accident deaths per year (McDonald, Lancet 1998) the estimated figure for total benzodiazepine-related deaths rises to around 17,000. According to Home Office 1990–1996 figures, benzodiazepine-related deaths exceed the number of deaths attributed to all Class A drugs put together.
> I understand that the Home Office is unable to provide figures for benzodiazepine-related deaths after 1996 because of a revised method of recording."

These statistics show a bleak picture. In Scotland in 1998, which is the most recent year figures are available for, 114 people died from heroin and morphine overdoses. But 151 died from taking benzodiazepines. In England and Wales between 1990 and 1996, 1,623 people overdosed on heroin, morphine and other opiates while 1,810 died from benzodiazepines.

Independent commentators and watchdogs can appreciate the real world situation as it applies to the consequences of prescriptions and their aftermath, but it seems that government watchdogs and government itself find it a little more difficult. For them, reality is in fact so hard to divine that black becomes white and regrettably, smoke obscures the facts. This Press release was issued by the independent NHS watchdog for London in 2003. What it had to say about London, it could have said about the entire UK, if that had been within its remit.

DOUBLE FAILURE FOR TRANQUILLISER DEPENDENT PATIENTS
London Health Link, August 11 2003

> London Health Link, the independent watchdog on London's NHS has produced a report on the experiences of patients who have been prescribed tranquillisers by their family doctors over a long period and the consequences of their resulting dependence on these drugs. This report highlights the lack of help and support from the NHS for people who experience health problems when they are taken off these drugs. For fifteen years the Department of Health has been recommending that this group of tranquillisers (benzodiazepines) should only be prescribed for up to four weeks, yet many patients report much longer use.
> Benzodiazepines can be highly addictive and the National Treatment Agency for Substance Misuse has stated: "They have strong addictive potential, the withdrawal syndrome can

be dangerous, and they are known to be a major contributor to deaths from drug misuse. Yet currently there are:
No NHS guidelines on withdrawal from long-term use,
No guidance on what services should be available to people who report problems AND
No NHS ownership of this problem.

London Health Link is calling for:
Compulsory Guidance to the NHS to help patients get off benzodiazepines
Monitoring to make sure that the NHS follows the Guidance
Services for people who experience problems from long-term benzodiazepine use

Elizabeth Manero, Chair of London Health Link, said:
"These patients have been doubly let down by the NHS. First they have been prescribed these drugs for far too long and become dependent. Secondly the NHS is failing to provide services to them to cope with that dependency. We are calling for this double failure to be addressed properly because we feel that this patient group has been totally neglected."

The Nature of the Beast

"Almost two decades of laissez faire research [into diazepam, chlordiazepoxide and meprobamate] have yielded no systematic base data for meaningful inferences...Surely this deplorable net result of undirected and misdirected science and pseudo-science suggests that some routine should be established to provide a comparative data base for evaluating the effects on performance of any anti-anxiety drug marketed for administration to humans."
McNair DM: Antianxiety drugs and human performance; Arch Gen Psychiatry, November **1983**, 29,611–7

"I don't think anyone really knows what long-term effects the benzodiazepines are likely to have on the brain tissue, [they] may damage your brain cells and produce real physical damage to your thinking processes and there is also the risk that the benzodiazepines will cause psychological damage."
Dr Vernon Coleman, 'Life Without Tranquillisers', **1985**

"Sternbach never understood the fuss. Now 91, he retired in 1973 with over 230 patents to his name; La Roche paid him a piddling $10,000 a year for 10 years to reward him for Valium.
usnews.com, December 27 **1999**

Benzodiazepine and other Drug Realities

Benzodiazepines are much more than a question of harm done by the medical profession. There is also the central question of each successive government, nominally overseeing the health service, allowing them to do it. Government and medical dismissal of patient experience as relatively minor and short-term is nothing more than a hierarchical repetition of false assertions, the original source of which (if it was ever known), has been lost.

What cannot be rationally doubted by the open-minded, is the fact that benzodiazepines are frequently seriously damaging—something which might not be immediately apparent, judging by the truly enormous quantities that doctors have prescribed over the years, both in the UK and in other countries. There were warnings from very early in the life of these drugs that this was so, but the drug companies successfully fought off the findings for nearly thirty years until benzodiazepines were old news.

The primary effect of benzodiazepines is one of addiction. With regular use for only a few months or even weeks the body comes to depend on them both psychologically and physically for normal functioning. As a consequence of this dependence, tolerance develops, so that larger doses are needed to produce the same initial effects. There is clear evidence showing that hypnotic effects are no longer effective after a few weeks and anxiolytic effects after only a few months. People unknowingly continue taking them mainly to prevent withdrawal effects. If dosage is insufficient once tolerance has developed, or if the drug is completely stopped, withdrawal symptoms then develop. This is an important reason why the long-term prescribed feel so ill all the time. The Department of Health stubbornly and perversely ignores this basic scientific truth and has illogically introduced an instalment prescription plan. Quite how doling out prescriptions over days will benefit addicted patients is a question it refuses to answer. It looks like action and to government that is probably enough of a recommendation, but doctors tempted to give it a try, may well find the 'problem' becoming much more noticeable in their surgeries as a result.

At present there are over a million long-term prescribed benzodiazepine users in the UK. Several studies, including those carried out by Newcastle University, have shown from computerised prescribing records, that there are 180 or so such patients in every GP practice. These long-term patients, while continuing their drug use, often suffer from adverse effects and from withdrawal effects afterwards. Long-term use is commonly accompanied by increasingly diverse illnesses.

Professor C.H. Ashton, unlike those who advise government behind the scenes, ran an effective benzodiazepine withdrawal clinic from 1982–1994 at Newcastle University. She has described the morbidity in the first 50 consecutive patients who then attended. They had been taking prescribed "therapeutic" doses of benzodiazepines for between five and twenty years and had decided to withdraw because they did not feel well while taking the drugs. Of these, 20% suffered from agoraphobia and/or panic attacks, 10% had had neurological investigations (three for Multiple Sclerosis) and 18% had had gastrointestinal investigations. Backing up the argument that long-term benzodiazepines lead to other prescriptions, she said that 62% of the first group had been prescribed other psychotropic drugs since starting benzodiazepines, the most common being antidepressants. In addition, 28% had been prescribed two benzodiazepines, thereby doubling the addiction potential and the possibility of side-effects.

Professor Ashton has said categorically that the symptoms which led to the investigations and the polypharmacy, were not the reason for starting benzodiazepines, **but developed during long-term use**. She has said on several occasions, that there is a likelihood that health for everyone does not necessarily return to normal after prescriptions cease. In 2003 for example, she said:

> "Withdrawal symptoms can last months or years in fifteen percent of long-term users. In some people chronic use has resulted in long-term, possibly permanent disability."

In the Comprehensive Handbook of Drug & Alcohol Addiction 2004, she said:

> "For some chronic benzodiazepine users, withdrawal can be a long, drawn-out process. A sizeable minority (perhaps 10 to 15%) develop a "post-withdrawal syndrome" which may linger for months or even years."

From the current evidence it appears that the symptoms that are most likely to be long-lasting are anxiety and insomnia, cognitive impairment, depression, various sensory and motor phenomena, and gastrointestinal problems.

It may be that the anxiety which persists after the acute phase of withdrawal could be due in part to a range of learning defects caused by benzodiazepines. Tranquilliser drugs undoubtedly cause thought deficits and impair coping abilities. There may be an extended period after the taking of benzodiazepines has ceased when former patients find stressful situations difficult to deal with, though of course many still taking the drugs have the same experience as well. Something as basic as queuing in a shop, or answering the phone, can often seem a frightening and stressful situation. Complete recovery may require the individual to learn new strategies to replace the years of coping through drugs. For some people whose economic and social circumstances, have been severely impacted, this learning may prove to be inordinately difficult and sometimes impossible.

On any patient leaflet you will find advice saying that anxiety occurring after withdrawal is due to pre-existing symptoms recurring. Indeed it is normally cited by the profession as a reason why most doctors continue prescriptions. Patients who were not prescribed the drugs for clinical anxiety (and that is the majority) know that the self-serving 'symptoms recurring argument' is untrue. Professor Ashton has said:

> "...persistence or worsening of anxiety after withdrawal does not necessarily imply the re-emergence of an anxiety state existing before withdrawal. Indeed, some patients experience major panic attacks and agoraphobia for the first time after withdrawal and may, for a time, develop a more severe degree

> of anxiety than was present when the drugs were first prescribed..."

This can be a Catch 22 situation. Depression is common in long-term benzodiazepine users and patient experience points to the drugs being the cause. Depression also appears when patients withdraw. There may be pharmacological reasons for this but who would not be depressed by the realisation of what had been done to them by what they thought was a safe medicine? Depressive symptoms may appear for the very first time after withdrawal—often some weeks later, and may be severe and protracted for a long time. Suicide has been reported in some studies. Government maintains a supreme indifference to this benzodiazepine research. Instead it continues a parrot-like repetition of the need to prevent addiction occurring in the first place, ignoring the plight of many thousands of people disabled through medical prescribing.

Professor Malcolm Lader of the well-respected and influential London Institute of Psychiatry, has published more than a hundred papers on the subject of benzodiazepines over the years. In the BBC Radio 4 programme, 'Face the Facts' he said:

> "It is more difficult to withdraw people from benzodiazepines than it is from heroin. It just seems that the dependency is so ingrained and the withdrawal symptoms you get are so intolerable that people have a great deal of problem coming off. The other aspect is that with heroin, usually the withdrawal is over within one week or so. With the benzodiazepines, a proportion of patients go on to long-term withdrawal and they have very unpleasant symptoms for month after month, and I get letters from people saying you can go on for two years or more. Some of the tranquilliser groups can document people who still have symptoms ten years after stopping."

It may be difficult to believe that members of a still highly regarded profession, ostensibly dedicated to the improvement of health, could inflict such damage, but the fact is that most doctors have an affinity with potions, and with the rise of drug company influence, they developed an affinity with the manufacturers of them. The Director of the Promis Recovery Centre in Kent, Dr Robert Lefever, illustrated this fact well when he said:

> "Doctors prescribe by nature. I had a patient who told me that her doctor had warned her that if she came off her medication she might die. I just saw another patient who was on seventy tablets a day. There are doctors out there who are absolutely

> committed to prescribing, and if the patient doesn't get better, they just up the dose."

It was the psychopharmacalogical era beginning in the late fifties that led to the explosion of medically-induced ill health. Benzodiazepines were pushed by their manufacturers as appropriate for virtually anything. An advert for the first benzodiazepine Librium (chlordiazepoxide) was headed: 'Whatever the Diagnosis'. Doctors certainly took that message to heart, prescribing Librium and its successors for nearly every complaint under the sun. They followed the logic of the advert religiously:

> "In the face of ill health there is anxiety and where there is anxiety either as a complicating factor or as a cause of illness itself, there is a place for LIBRIUM."

Today, in spite of this reality, the UK Department of Health rigidly maintains an illusion that the drugs were normally prescribed for clinical anxiety and therefore suffering patients fall within the psychiatric sphere of responsibility. That way, it can say that any psychological problems while taking benzodiazepines or following withdrawal, are due to pre-prescription symptoms returning. They will not engage with the fact that patients, who were given the drugs for other reasons, are as likely to experience the same psychological difficulties as those who were given them for clinical anxiety. As Dr Ian Telfer, a consultant psychiatrist in the North of England said in 2000:

> "When they first came out they were seen as some sort of panacea—or universal remedy. But with constant use it was found they turned people into zombies in the end."

It has been claimed that benzodiazepines are the most researched drugs in the world but much of the early research was basic and superficial to say the least, and would not meet even today's standards. Long-term research has never taken place, either then or subsequently. Patients who took the drugs for years—many for decades—therefore have their claims of health damage, ignored and rejected in the face of zero scientific evidence that it did not happen. Professor Heather Ashton applied for research grants to explore the claims of long-term health damage in both 1995 and 1996, but her applications were unsuccessful. Possibly the authorities controlling research grants thought there were more important things to investigate or perhaps they believed there was existing research that obviated the need for investigation. Neither was true.

There are people who have taken the drugs and claim to have experienced no untoward effects or problems during ingestion or in withdrawal. I have no evidence to doubt that this can happen, but there are factors worth mentioning as to why this might be so. On the one side of the argument about the benefit of benzodiazepines and possible symptoms, there are psychiatrists such as Professor David Nutt at Bristol University, who believes the downside of benzodiazepines has been over-emphasised and that psychiatrists are being unduly limited in their use. In a May 2004 presentation entitled 'The Development of New Benzodiazepine (BDZ) and Other Sedative-Anxiolytic-Hypnotic (SAH) Guidelines Suitable for Use by General Adult Psychiatrists', he emphasised that benzodiazepine withdrawal reactions take a long time to develop:

"4 weeks: very low risk
4 months: 5–10%
2 years: 25–45%
6–8 years: 75%"

But this is far from being the definitive picture. There **is** a correlation between length of use and symptoms, but there are many other factors involved, for example dose levels, the type of benzodiazepine used, the reasons for the initial prescription, the personality of the patients and so on. Moreover it has been clearly demonstrated that withdrawal symptoms (e.g. sleep symptoms) can occur after as little as one week of drug use. Dr Anthony Kales, and others in Pennsylvania, produced clear evidence of this happening. Trying to quantify the incidence of addiction and withdrawal reaction, therefore involves much more than simple length of use, even if long-term use is an important factor.

Professor Heather Ashton agrees that some people can withdraw from benzodiazepines with few if any symptoms and that there are probably many reasons why. Personality may play a part and this ultimately has a physical basis, shaped by genetics and environment which determines the "wiring up" of the brain—e.g. the synaptic connections which mediate the ways that individuals have learnt to cope with anxiety and stress. There is evidence that anxious people have fewer GABA/benzodiazepine receptors in the emotional areas of the brain than more stolid people—so perhaps those without withdrawal symptoms had more GABA receptors to utilise. They may not develop so much benzodiazepine tolerance (down-regulation of GABA/benzodiazepine receptors) and so suffer less rebound of GABA under activity related to withdrawal symptoms. The distribution and sensitivity of these receptors may vary so that some people may have more physical symptoms in withdrawal while others experience more psychological symptoms.

The nature of withdrawal may, she says, depend partly on the type of benzodiazepine used. Withdrawal symptoms are usually worse in those using short-acting and/or potent benzodiazepines such as lorazepam, alprazolam, and clonazepam even if these are withdrawn slowly. The rate of withdrawal obviously also plays a part. Some people with severe symptoms have withdrawn too quickly, have been switched to another benzodiazepine of less equivalent potency or have had previous traumatic "cold turkey" experiences. Some patients actually develop a type of post-traumatic stress disorder (PTSD) giving them a fear of withdrawal. Fear and expectation can play a large part in how withdrawal goes, she believes—no advance fears mean there are no negative expectations and therefore a greater possibility of no symptoms. On the other hand, as she admits, there are others who are taken by surprise by withdrawal symptoms they did not expect. Her estimate of symptom-less withdrawal in the general population is around ten percent. However careful the dosage reduction some patients dependent on benzodiazepines may develop symptoms.

A crucial ingredient, seldom if ever, ever mentioned in relation to benzodiazepine withdrawal, is the factor of polypharmacy, which Professor Ashton agrees may well play a part. She says that over 60% of the long-term dependent she saw in her National Health Service Withdrawal Clinic, had also been prescribed other drugs, usually antidepressants, along with the benzodiazepines. Antidepressants, antipsychotics, and morphine-based painkillers, all have side-effects themselves—with symptoms not completely dissimilar to benzodiazepine withdrawal. It is for this reason that she has always suggested that people stay on their antidepressants until they have finished benzodiazepine withdrawal. In that way they do not experience a multiple withdrawal syndrome. Any discussion by anyone on the subject of benzodiazepine withdrawal is therefore necessarily incomplete, if it does not take into account the fact that for many people, benzodiazepine prescriptions led to other drug prescriptions—many of them producing physical dependence. It is often a situation of withdrawing from multi-drug use, rather than single drug use.

So, the experience of people who have taken (or who are still taking) benzodiazepines and indeed other psychiatric drugs, varies. There are a number of reasons for the individuality of response, not least, differences in human physical make-up, length of prescription and differences in personal circumstances. A person working in a job, which does not require high-level intellectual thought, or constant decision-making, for instance, may find it altogether easier to avoid the impact of benzodiazepines on cognition.

Some people claim to find benzodiazepines, Z drugs (zopiclone, zaleplon and others) or SSRIs, helpful or essential for dealing with their lives, and the purpose of this book is not to convince them otherwise. The purpose of this book is to represent the tens of thousands whose experience has been quite different (including the many thousands who have died), and seeks to provide a contextual analysis of why medicine damages in the way it does and why the providers of medicine and its regulators maintain a message of safety when clearly it is not true. Some people taking psychotropic prescriptions may be willing to endure unwanted side-effects of the drugs they take for the sake of perceived benefit, but far more likely is a situation where, in the absence of information, they continue to take the drugs without linking the decline in their health to their medicine.

There needs to be some sort of true representation for the stories of the very large numbers of UK citizens whose existence has been needlessly harmed and sometimes destroyed by prescribed benzodiazepine addiction. Benzodiazepines are not the only drugs to destroy health and lives and there are strong common elements between the stories of different drugs —pharmaceutical company deceit, regulatory inaction, and dogged medical belief in benefit, is common to all. But it is the scale of benzodiazepine prescribing and its longevity that makes this story unique. Benzodiazepines have been prescribed in their hundreds of millions to millions of patients, based on a jigsaw of poor and non-existent research, pharmaceutical power, amateur regulation, medical ignorance and disdain, and organised government cover-up.

We live in a society which has been largely indoctrinated by the pharmaceutical industry, and by the medical profession which it educates— into the belief that psychiatric drugs are safe and effective and properly prescribed. None of these things is ultimately true. Any media examination of the downside of a particular drug is, (as a reassurance), almost always accompanied by an unsubstantiated statement that millions have been helped. This message comes straight from the pharmaceutical industry but because of the widespread belief in society in drug safety and effectiveness, and the power of science, it is duly reported as fact, without questioning or analysis.

How are statistics of large benefit and little harm arrived at? What rigorous investigation is it based on? Is it, for instance, based on the absence of complaint to doctors, regulators or drug companies? Is it based on collected endorsements from patients? Or is based on neither of these? Is it, in fact, not a statistic at all—merely another plank in the house built by the indoctrinators? But the desire to believe is strong. It is a sad but observable fact that we look beyond positive claims and assurances only after we have personally met the hidden downside of drugs that 'help millions', through our own experience.

The question that is never asked or answered is why patient evidence is invariably marginalised or disbelieved in medicine—by doctors and by those whose job description is the protection of public health from drug harm. A doctor accepts what the patient says before he makes a decision to prescribe a drug. Why does he invariably disbelieve complaints afterwards about the effects of the drug? In psychotropic medicine, the answer to that question is simple. Once you have accepted a prescription for a mind altering drug, you are no longer a reliable reporter—you are in fact, a mental patient—even if what you were given the drug for has less to do with 'mental disease' and a great deal more to do with the pressures surrounding individuals in society. The fact that someone is given a psychotropic prescription, means in Western society, that everything they say thereafter, is unreliable and questionable. This is the stranglehold that psychotropic drugs and their producers have over medicine and the individuals in society.

Social and general costs of iatrogenic benzodiazepine addiction

Benzodiazepines have been a near 50 year horror story for tens of thousands of people in the UK but this medical disgrace has never been addressed. Weak, belated and spasmodic warnings have been issued over the years and they have had the unfortunate side-effect for patients, of allowing government and the benzodiazepine manufacturers to further draw a veil over the historic and ongoing impact of inappropriate prescribing in the public mind.

It is possible to make an argument that much of the medical profession does not fully realise what it has done, given the speed of consultations, the failure of regulators to pass on the horror stories they have been told, and the distance between the patient in the doctor's surgery and the patient's actual life outside it. But above all, it is the chemical ability of benzodiazepines to produce apparent mental instability and engender a belief, not only in doctors but also in patients, that this drug-produced harm is genuine illness that has led to the greatest medical damage. The belief has been fostered among doctors (and often the patients), that the drugs and consequent ones have been necessary.

It is far from true that benzodiazepine injury (called a scandal by some), has ever been addressed in any way that patients would find meaningful. There are still far too many prescribed addicts in the UK and thousands of former addicts who took the drugs long-term, and as a result are living with ruined health which cannot be rebuilt. Many are living in poverty because of the effects of benzodiazepines. Whole lives have been lost and cannot be relived. Families have disintegrated, never to reunite.

The real severity of benzodiazepine damage has never been officially recognised. In the face of it the Department of Health maintains a belief that benzodiazepine addiction is not all that serious and withdrawal is relatively easy. In modern government-speak the department 'does not recognise' the experience related by affected patients or campaigners. The Department too believes that repeated utterance of statements such as 'we take the problem seriously' or 'our priority is to prevent addiction occurring in the first place' makes it true for actual and former patients and is adequate support for those badly in need of it.

The debate on benzodiazepines has largely centred on addiction versus efficacy, but addiction can be seen as only part of the picture—mostly important in its relation to the fact that once addicted, patients keep taking them. The far more serious side of the issue centres around what continued addiction often leads to, and its dire effects on general health, thinking abilities, and life.

There are extensive costs to the patient and to society, caused by benzodiazepines but not studied by medicine, because their nature is not seen as medical. There are costs produced by benzodiazepines which are medical but which have never been researched, and which are therefore not recognised by medicine

There are costs to the National Health Service for example, of medical investigations for symptoms which are in reality a result of the effects of benzodiazepines. These costs must be very high indeed, if patient reporting is taken into account, but they are officially unquantified. Investigations for MS, ME, IBS, Arthritis and Thyroid deficiency and other 'ghost illnesses' are common—usually the results are negative.

For people taking benzodiazepines and particularly the elderly, there is a much increased risk of accidents. The cause of the accidents, whether occurring in the home, on the road, at work or in a care home is routinely not recognised, but has a cost for the individual beyond the cost to the NHS.

There is a great deal of evidence that the unborn are severely affected by the addiction of the mother. The link between benzodiazepines and foetal harm was denied in Parliament in 1999 but it undoubtedly occurs. This raises the serious question of why it was denied. Readers can consult Sue Bibby's site at www.benzact.org.uk

Between the introduction of benzodiazepines and 2004, Home Office and other figures suggest 17,000 deaths associated with benzodiazepines but as with all official statistics, they may well be an underestimate. In reply to a question from the Parliamentary Health Committee in 2004, Professor Alasdair Breckenridge, the Chairman of the UK drugs regulator stated that he thought there had been approximately 170 deaths. As Professor Heather Ashton said at the time, this represented 1% of the total and was a gross under-representation on the part of the regulator.

Prescribed benzodiazepines can lead to loss of control over actions which means in practice that drug-induced violence occurs in the home involving partners and children. Unwanted pregnancies are another side-effect of the drugs. Inhibition reduction leads to anti-social acts such as theft and vandalism. Benzodiazepines cause job loss either whilst taking them or while attempting to withdraw. Not everyone loses their job of course but a significantly large number do, and it is not surprising, given the deadening effects of the addiction and the high number and severity of possible withdrawal effects. This effect on the individual and on families is totally ignored by government. In 2004 the Chief Medical Officer, Professor Liam Donaldson, reminded doctors of their continuing over-prescribing. He referred to the cost to the NHS of the drugs themselves, but made no mention of the costs to the individual.

There is a large financial impact to the state generally, which benzodiazepine addiction is responsible for. People who are unable to work pay no taxes or national insurance. Their spending power is curtailed and therefore they pay less VAT. Addicted and unemployed the benzodiazepine-dependent make very little contribution to the economy. Although many iatrogenic benzodiazepine addicts are to all intents and purposes disabled, few receive disability benefits. Thousands do receive incapacity benefit at a lower figure, because of the length of their 'illness', and this is of course a drain on the national economy. Many iatrogenic victims have not worked for decades.

Perhaps the biggest loss for a proportion of the dependent (and who knows how big this proportion is) is the loss of choice. They cannot choose to buy a house or might lose a house because of the drug effects. They cannot take holidays or buy a new car. They cannot socialise or take up hobbies because of induced anxiety and inability to concentrate. Some discover after they have withdrawn from the drugs that they never left the house or indeed a room, for years because of benzo agoraphobia—prisoners because of drug prescriptions.

There is much exhortation from government these days about the need to build up personal pensions to maintain a secure lifestyle in retirement—we are all living longer and the state is becoming more hard-pressed to finance pensioners it seems. There are thousands, addicted for decades to benzodiazepines, who feel assaulted anew when they hear that message. Through state avoidance of responsibility for health protection, they had no chance to build up a personal pension, leaving them entirely dependent on the state for the future. What a supreme irony it is then, that at a time when the state is telling everyone that the state pension is completely inadequate and that they should save for a personal one, there are many condemned to poverty through state inactivity and denial.

The most insidious effect of the drugs in the estimation of many is the effect the drugs have had on their family. The family was not prescribed the drugs but it was as certainly and indelibly marked as the taker. The lack of emotional response due to benzodiazepines is something a child does not understand and may never understand, even as an adult. The life chances of children of the unemployed and sick iatrogenic addict are necessarily reduced and their emotional needs may remain unsatisfied, leading to problems for them later in life. It can be very difficult afterwards to re-establish relationships between a formerly addicted parent and children.

Additionally, Professor Heather Ashton has in various lectures referred to the incidence of mortality from overdose, suicide and accidents. At a Benzodiazepine Conference in Oldham in 2004 she said:

> "A recent study estimated that benzodiazepines cause 1600 traffic accidents and 110 driving-related deaths each year in the UK."
>
> "Between1990–1996, over 1800 deaths have been attributed to benzodiazepine overdose in suicides, accidents and undetermined causes. In about two thirds of these cases, benzodiazepines were taken alone; in one third with alcohol or other drugs. Benzodiazepines are taken in 40% of self-poisonings. Temazepam, the commonest hypnotic used today, is the most toxic. The risk of a fatal outcome is greatly increased in the elderly and people with lung disease, and benzodiazepines increase the risk of fatality if taken with many other drugs that depress respiration. The combination of benzodiazepines with opiates causes about 100 deaths each year among drug abusers in Glasgow alone."
> Professor Heather Ashton

Benzodiazepines might well help some people in the short-term, owing to their properties as hypnotics, anticonvulsants, muscle relaxants, amnesics and anxiolytics. But benzodiazepines have incredibly serious potential adverse effects made even worse by polypharmacy, excessive dosages and long-term use. Benzodiazepines were largely sold to doctors as being much less toxic than their predecessors the barbiturates but they are a long way from being safe drugs. High doses of benzodiazepines lead to over-sedation. The symptoms include poor concentration, mental confusion, muscle weakness and impaired balance and co-ordination. These symptoms can carry over into the next day, particularly with long-acting benzodiazepines such as nitrazepam (Mogadon) and diazepam (Valium). The elderly, as can be imagined, are the most vulnerable, but younger people are not immune.

Benzodiazepines impact on the ability to think, make decisions, and to remember. They make it much harder to learn new information. There are people who have withdrawn from benzodiazepines who find they have lost whole years and decades of their lives. In the elderly, these effects can lead to a false diagnosis of Alzheimer's disease. In spite of this fact, many occupants of old people's homes and in the community are regularly prescribed benzodiazepines. As Professor Ashton says:

> "Benzodiazepines can occasionally cause paradoxical aggression and have been associated with baby-battering, wife-beating and grandma-bashing. They can also cause depression and can precipitate suicide in depressed patients. They should not be used in depression although they are still commonly prescribed long-term for depressed and anxious patients. They can also cause emotional blunting and apathy, with inability to cope with the needs of children and family, an effect bitterly regretted by many long-term users."

Perhaps the most innocent in this story of widespread harm for the innocent, are pregnant mothers and the new-born. If taken regularly during pregnancy, benzodiazepines can cause adverse effects on the foetus and neonate and may possibly contribute to cot deaths since the neonate is unable to metabolise them efficiently. But they are still prescribed during pregnancy.

Where does the patient find closure in the face of orchestrated denial, lack of government recognition and help, and a spirit within the medical profession that sees each new drug as a wonder drug, taking decades each time before it exercises control? The three components of continuing good health are psychological, physical and social. Benzodiazepines have a three-pronged negative effect on health—the effects of taking them, the realisation afterwards of the impact they had on a life and the realisation for the individual that they are powerless to achieve recognition. It is a deep and genuine kind of grief which is not in the annals of medicine. Within the present political, legal and medical structures, there is little hope of closure.

The Commentators

> "The risks of these drugs [benzodiazepines] often outweigh therapeutic benefits."
> Health Canada, 1996 Review of Benzodiazepine Use

> "The world's biggest addiction problem is not teenagers taking hash but middle-agers taking sedatives. The tranquilliser is replacing tobacco. It will, perhaps, give us an even bigger problem. It may prove even more dangerous. Already Valium is said to be taken by 14% of the population of Britain. The habit usually starts insidiously. The patient may have a good

excuse for taking a few tablets. A close friend or relative has died or there is a rush on at work. And the doctor finds it difficult to refuse the request for a little help. The drugs which people take to help relieve their pressures vary. If he is young the addict may take drugs from a pusher. If he is older he may take drugs from a medical adviser."
Dr Vernon Coleman, 'The Medicine Men' 1975

"The medical profession took nearly 20 years from the introduction of benzodiazepines to recognise officially that these minor tranquillisers and hypnotics were potentially addictive. The 'happiness pills', which had been propping up a fair proportion of the adult population since the early 1960s, were found to have an unexpectedly bitter aftertaste: doctors and patients alike were unprepared for the problems of dependence and withdrawal that are now known to be common even with normal therapeutic doses."
Editorial (Anon), The Benzodiazepine Bind, The Lancet, 22 September 1984, 706

"There's certainly a problem, the NHS are concerned. The NHS spends about £40 million per annum on these drugs. There are a substantial number of people who do suffer from this problem long-term. I know that the withdrawal symptoms can be agonising for some people and can be very difficult indeed."
John Patten, Health Minister, 1984

"And then the alarm bells started to ring, quietly at first and then louder and louder...Doctors were not well equipped to deal with this. This was something new in their experience. They don't like dealing with chronic drug use or addiction anyway and here they were being confronted by hundreds in their practices—who they had put on the tranquillisers—and were now coming for help to come off. And I think they were bewildered by the numbers and severity of some of the reactions...The main characteristic of these dependent people was that when they tried to stop they didn't just get their old symptoms back, they didn't just get their old symptoms back in an exaggerated form, they developed new symptoms which they had not experienced before...Some people are put on to these tranquillisers not because they are anxious or have insomnia, they can't sleep...and they're put on and they've had no psychiatric history, they've had no anxiety, no insomnia,

and yet they're just as likely to show dependence and withdrawal when they stop as those with a previous psychiatric history."
Professor Malcolm H. Lader, Institute of Psychiatry, 'In Pills We Trust', Discovery Channel, December 2002

"Benzos are responsible for more pain, unhappiness and damage than anything else in our society."
Phil Woolas MP, Deputy Leader of the House of Commons and Local Government Minister, Oldham Chronicle, February 12 2004

"The Medical profession, I think, is fairly ashamed of what has happened. It has allowed this very untrammelled prescribing to go on. My estimate is that there's something between a quarter and half a million people in this country, at this moment, who would have problems trying to stop their tranquillisers. They would need help to do so and there's been a sense that they're difficult to treat, difficult to deal with and a lot of these patients are just kept on their medication indefinitely. No real attempt is made to help them come off...The Government should tackle this problem face on. There are thousands of people out there who are not receiving treatment, hundreds of GPs who don't know really how to treat these patients. There are self-help groups who are crying out for funding just to keep going at a very low level. I think the Government should now acknowledge the problem and set funds aside, because if the Government doesn't do that, these people will go to their graves with their tranquilliser bottles beside them."
Professor Malcolm H. Lader, 'Face the Facts', BBC Radio 4 1991

"Some people have been on benzodiazepines for many years, and it is very difficult to get them off because they are very addictive."
Peter Fellows, Chairman of the British Medical Association's Prescribing Committee, BBC News, February 11 2004

"Physical and psychological dependence on tranquillisers can happen in an alarmingly short space of time. You reach a stage where you can't cope without tranquillisers and are terrified of trying to stop taking them...Suffering withdrawal from tranquillisers is no joke, but it can be done. Those who

have gone through it say that it must be harder than coming off heroin."
Dr Miriam Stoppard, Broadcaster and Writer, 2005

"Doctors who prescribe benzodiazepines continuously are courting disaster. What we need to realize is that benzodiazepines are addictive...The drugs should not generally be prescribed for longer than a few weeks. You use them clinically when it is indicated for short periods of time. Short-term use is certainly less than three months. In general practice I wouldn't be using them for more than two to three weeks...It is a drug that takes a much longer detox procedure than almost anything else"
Drug-addictions expert Dr. Garth McIver, The Vancouver Province, December 31 2001

"There's still a significant continuing problem with benzodiazepines in this country. We would have liked if it was solved 20 years ago, but it still exists. We continue to work as a College with prescribing groups around the country to try and continue to raise awareness of this issue and reduce the prescribing of these drugs to appropriate use, but it is a very long struggle...I think it should be a significant priority for this country. It's potentially a million people who are on drugs which only maybe is a tiny percentage of them need to be on, and that is not good for this country. It's also a waste of resource. We are ploughing money into these drugs and into support services for patients for a situation that we may have created ourselves."
Dr Jim Kennedy, Royal College of General Practitioners, 'The Tranquilliser Trap', BBC, May 2001

"It is difficult to defend that we have such a huge problem of benzodiazepine prescription and long-term use and therefore dependence."
Professor Louis Appleby, National Director for Mental Health, 'The Tranquilliser Trap', BBC, May 2001

"If the popular press and more recently the legal profession had not taken up arms against the over prescription of tranquillisers, the issue of benzodiazepine dependence would still remain a medical curio only for the pages of medical journals. The media and lawyers have undoubtedly altered prescribing practices mostly for the better."

Dr Cosmo Hallström, Journal of Forensic Psychiatry 1991

"Benzodiazepine dependence would be of minor clinical significance if it occurred only in those few individuals taking high doses of drugs; but it would be very important indeed if it supervened even to a minor degree in patients on usual clinical doses. Our clinical impression is that many patients experience symptoms on reduction or withdrawal of their benzodiazepine medication, and that whilst these symptoms somewhat resemble those of anxiety they differ qualitatively and are often more severe than those for which the medication was originally given."
Hallström and Lader, Benzodiazepine withdrawal phenomena, Int. Pharmacopsychiatry, 1981, 16, 235–244

"The benzodiazepines are probably the most addictive drugs ever created and the vast army of enthusiastic doctors who prescribed these drugs by the tonne have created the world's largest drug addiction problem."
Dr Vernon Coleman, 'The Drugs Myth', 1992

"In the UK, 11.2% of all adults take an anti-anxiety drug at some time during any one year. But over a quarter of these people (3.1% of all adults) are chronic users, taking such medication every day. Even at a conservative estimate, 20% of these will develop symptoms when they attempt to withdraw. That means a quarter of a million people in the UK. The sooner the medical profession faces up to its responsibilities towards these iatrogenic addicts, the sooner it will regain the confidence of the anxious members of our community."
M.H. Lader, Anna C. Higgitt, Management of benzodiazepine dependence, Update 1986, Brit J Addiction, 1986, 81, 7–10

"It has been estimated that one in three patients, prescribed benzodiazepines in normal therapeutic doses for six weeks, would experience withdrawal symptoms if treatment were withdrawn abruptly. Even with gradual withdrawal, patients would request further prescriptions. Thus, there is a considerable risk of dependence even in comparatively short-term use."
M.A. Cormack, R.G. Owens, M.E. Dewey, The effect of minimal interventions by general practitioners on long-term

benzodiazepines use, Journal of Royal College of General Practitioners, October 1989, 39, 408–411

"People were innocently put on this medication [Xanax] and in some instances it works out well. [But] there is a significant risk and we see it all of the time. Many people who have lost many years of their lives, who have lost jobs, been on the verge of suicide. I'm aware of cases where people have committed suicide. The drug can be dangerous, it can be fatal. During withdrawal the heart rate can go up, they may have a seizure, sometimes the body temperature can go up and in some instances it's fatal."
Dr. Neil Capretto, Director of the Gateway Rehabilitation Centre in Pennsylvania.

"The biggest drug-addiction problem in the world doesn't involve heroin, cocaine or marijuana. In fact, it doesn't involve an illegal drug at all. The world's biggest drug-addiction problem is posed by a group of drugs, the benzodiazepines, which are widely prescribed by doctors and taken by countless millions of perfectly ordinary people around the world...Drug-addiction experts claim that getting people off the benzodiazepines is more difficult than getting addicts off heroin...For several years now pressure-groups have been fighting to help addicted individuals break free from their pharmacological chains. But the fight has been a forlorn one. As fast as one individual breaks free from one of the benzodiazepines, another patient somewhere else becomes addicted."
Dr Vernon Coleman,' Life Without Tranquillisers', 1985

They [benzodiazepines] are very effective at relieving anxiety, but we now know that they can be addictive after only four weeks regular use. When people try to stop taking them they may experience unpleasant withdrawal symptoms which can go on for some time. These drugs should be only used for short periods, perhaps to help during a crisis. They should not be used for longer-term treatment of anxiety.
The Royal College of Psychiatrists, July 2001

"Benzodiazepines cause a more significant withdrawal for the newborn baby than either heroin or methadone. When a baby is withdrawing, they have a state of irritability, they are hyper-responsive, which means that they tremor at the slightest

noise, even when quiet and they cry with a cry that is very distinctive—it's much higher pitched and it's much more of a distressed cry as if the baby is in discomfort. They basically are miserable, unsettled babies."
Dr James Robertson, Arrowe Park Hospital, Liverpool, 'Face the Facts', BBC Radio 4, 1999

"The developing foetus can be congenitally malformed; it can have heart attacks in the womb. We also know that the newborn baby born to somebody taking benzodiazepines will have difficulty breathing and they would have floppy muscles—what doctors call a 'floppy baby' and they may be unduly cold because the temperature regulation, which is so important to a baby, is disrupted...Well I think if any doctor is prescribing benzodiazepines to a pregnant woman, he should check his indemnification status because it is in fact illegal prescribing."
Robert Kerwin, Professor of Psychopharmacology at the Maudesley Hospital in London, 'Face the Facts', BBC Radio 4 1999

"Amnesia is frequently a real side effect of the use of benzodiazepines and not just a figment of the individual's imagination or a coincident symptom of emotional disorder."
"It is recognised that the use of benzodiazepines has been (and is still) far too widespread and they are frequently prescribed for trivial and imprecise indications. This has arisen from the belief that benzodiazepines were safe compounds."
"It is now acknowledged that the risks of benzodiazepines far outweigh the benefits in many cases."
Priest RG, Montgomery SA. Benzodiazepines and Dependence: A College Statement. Bulletin of the Royal College of Psychiatrists 1988; 12:107–109

"We have much more difficulty getting people off Ativan than we do heroin, mainly because with heroin...within a couple of weeks they're off and then the problem is staying off. But with Ativan it's much more prolonged and they take up a lot more time in terms of treatment than do heroin users."
Jim Corcoran, Torbay Drug Addiction Team, 'Brass Tacks', BBC2, October 20 1987

"Thousands of people could not possibly invent the bizarre symptoms caused by therapeutic use of

benzodiazepines and reactions to their withdrawal. Many users have to cope, not only with a frightening range of symptoms, but also with the disbelief and hostility of their doctors and families. It is not uncommon for patients to be "struck off" if they continue to complain about withdrawal symptoms. Even when doctors are concerned and understanding about the problem, they often have little knowledge of withdrawal procedure, even less about treatment..." [My emphasis]

Trickett S, Withdrawal from Benzodiazepines, Journal of the Royal College of General Practitioners 1983; 33: 608

The Anointed

"It is a fantastic profession, a noble profession and if I could choose to start my life again, I would become a doctor."
John Hutton, Minister of State for Health at the British Medical Association Conference, September 2004

"The medical profession should take much responsibility for allowing the present situation to arise. They have been guilty of decades of thoughtless prescribing which persists for benzodiazepines despite national and international guidelines, recommending that benzodiazepines are indicated for short-term use [2–4 weeks] only."
Professor C. Heather Ashton DM, FRCP, Bristol and District Tranquilliser Project AGM, October 2005

"How the dependence potential of the benzodiazepines was overlooked by doctors...is a matter for amazement and casts shame on the medical profession which claims to be scientifically based."
Professor C.H. Ashton, ibid

"These patients taking prescribed benzodiazepines regularly for six months, a year, often many years, have become dependent on the drugs through no fault of their own, yet they receive little medical help or advice."
Professor C.H. Ashton, 'The Ashton Manual', 1999–2007

Prescribers of medicine are unique in society—they have the freedom from control enjoyed by an Art, but are defended (and defend themselves), by reference to the certainties of a Science. They took no part in the science and rely on reports of what the science demonstrates from pharmaceutical companies. Nevertheless they regard themselves as experts in the use of the science, as does the majority of the public. Once approved, drugs (the science in concrete form), appear to have a strange immunity to critical questions and most importantly, to patient reporting of the actual adverse events associated with them. Examine the evidence on drug harm closely enough, and you wonder why doctors inflict the degree of injury that they do through drugs and consistently deny that they do it.

> "In every branch of medicine, doctors have established a unique immunity to serious challenge—the 'I am God' syndrome, and many doctors really believe it."
> Marese Hudson, 'This is Madness' ed. Newnes, Holmes, Dunn, 1999

Official rejection of benzodiazepine damage and the move to forget it, goes beyond poor regulation, perverse prescribing by doctors and the isolation of patients from information. A political decision was made to carry out a policy of denial within the Department of Health. No other explanation fits the historical facts. Doctors have been the benefactors of this policy and patients the victims.

In early 1965, Dr Martin E. P. Seligman observed that after conducting electric shock tests on dogs a number of times, the dogs stopped jumping. Instead, they simply lay down and waited for the shock. They had given up hope. The psychologist realised that when a creature believes it has no control over its situation and that whatever it does is futile, it begins to believe it is helpless and stops trying to fight or escape. He termed this condition "learned helplessness". This is a tool understood and employed by successive governments. They have consistently said they are listening to benzodiazepine patients and take prescribed addiction seriously, but in fact they do little to change the situation, in the hope that campaigners will eventually give up, accepting there is nothing they can do to produce change.

Tranquilliser harm is still around because doctors remain uninformed and uncontrolled. It has not been addressed in any effective way for reasons of politics, because medicine has become in some ways a political arm of government. The DoH believes that if the drugs are controlled in a way which allows the consumer to know in advance just how serious their effects can be, doctors may be left with nothing to offer and the pharmaceutical industry will be adversely affected. Doctors do not understand that a large part of their time is taken up with dealing with what are unacknowledged drug effects. SSRIs purported to be a new generation of positive benefit compounds, non-addictive and with negligible side-effects. This was not true for tranquillisers and it is not true for SSRIs. To perpetuate the public belief in doctors and in medicines, the DoH has of necessity to deny and ignore harm. To provide cover for itself and for doctors, lip service is paid to the idea of patient protection. There are warnings and there is guidance, but the warnings are muted, circumspect, reverential and restricted. And guidelines are after all, only guidelines, as pointed out in the film 'Pirates of the Caribbean'. Nothing substitutes for clinical judgement in the world of medicine.

Benzodiazepines are sedative/hypnotics, depending on the dose and strength of the drug. The original sedative/hypnotics were alcohol and opium. For a long time opium was used as a treatment for alcoholism. The irony was that as both drugs were addictive, an individual could end up with two addictions rather than one. Today there are those in medicine who see nothing wrong with using benzodiazepines in the same way as opium, often leading to the same result. Today, because of the insidious nature of long-term benzodiazepine prescribing, there are patients who become not only addicted to tranquillisers—sometimes more than one, but also to painkillers and to antidepressants.

In 1857 bromides were introduced, as opium, alcohol and cocaine became less medically fashionable, followed by chloral hydrate in 1869. Chloral immediately became very popular indeed—being prescribed in millions of doses, a foreshadowing of the enthusiastic prescribing of hundreds of millions of benzodiazepine tablets and capsules. Bromides and chloral hydrate were followed by barbiturates, drugs which were deadly in overdose or when mixed with alcohol. There is a clear history here of the medical profession learning nothing, of not understanding what addiction is, and believing that each new drug represents the dawn of a new era. Each drug is introduced, is widely and ignorantly prescribed, and only long afterwards condemned. A new wonder drug is formulated and it all goes on as before. And over time, rejecting Hippocrates, doctors have become remarkably proficient at blaming the patient rather than themselves.

Doctors can damage or kill you with kindness; they can do it through indifference or through incompetence. Because of the degree of control pharmaceutical companies have over drug information and regulation, they also have a misguided personal belief that they are the reason for the existence of healthcare and not the patient. It is because doctors are a scarce resource that the first priority of government is also not the patient but the doctor. The process of deciding what to prescribe seems to go somewhat like this:

Step 1

Consult memory on information supplied by:

a) Drug company representative.
b) Drug company sponsored expert at drug company financed seminar.
c) Relevant drug company literature.
d) Drug company advertising in medical journal.
e) Drug company assessment of drug company conducted research.

Step 2

Prescribe drug then uppermost in mind.

Note: For definitive information on side-effects, mentally review all of the above and if time allows—which it normally will not—consult the drug company Summary of Product Characteristics.

Prescribers do not set out to do harm, but as a profession they include the incompetent and the uncaring and most find it easier to listen to the message coming from the drug companies rather than the patient. Many find it easiest to blame the patient for the negative health effects of their prescriptions. Most are pragmatists, politically naive and believers in a system which has a distinct air of fundamentalism about it. I have thought for some time that medicine has a great deal in common with religion and feudalism, and I have produced internet images, centred on state drug regulators existing in a Court of Screwed Medicine, within an ersatz church, a historic human power construct which once held the population in thrall. The prescribers of mind altering drugs have become a closet arm of government. The general acceptance of the 'expert' in society provides a working camouflage for what is going on. The stresses of modern life and their consequences have been medicalised, providing a huge income for those who provide 'treatments' for those consequences. Medicine and government feed off each other. Each supports the other. Medicine is the newly established religion in society. Not to believe in drug applications and their benefits is the new heresy. And as though written for the subject of drug benefit, author, screenwriter and historian, Len Deighton once said:

"There is no such thing as truth, just universally accepted lies."

If you look at allopathic medicine long enough, that conclusion is inescapable. It is not evidence-based medicine as far as prescribers and regulators are concerned, it is faith-based medicine, and like the priests of old, the uninitiated (and the initiated who dare question) are either cast out from the sanctuary of the mainstream, or exhorted to believe in a higher truth which only true believers have access to. Suffer the peasants not to question my judgement is the abiding creed. In politics, fundamentalism is condemned but in medicine it is the basis for maintaining the system. Just as church and state were the pillars of the establishment, now medicine and state join forces. Psychotropic medicine serves the same purpose as religion once did—it keeps the imaginative and the dispossessed parts of the population from examining society and the human condition too closely.

At the centre of it all, is the fact that 99% of the general population is ignorant of the wealth of evidence on drug damage, whether it be from benzodiazepines or more recent potentially harmful drugs such as SSRIs and antipsychotics. If they saw the evidence—being non-scientists, they would on the whole I think, accept it. Those who have to be convinced of the evidence therefore, are the 1% or so who are scientists, particularly those involved in lobbying groups or other vested interests, and it is a fact that scientists are a very difficult bunch to convince, mainly because their education brands most of them for life. Prescribers are the end-users of research they take no part in. They have no training in analysis of data and have little time to do it. Their world is dependent on the scientific message that drugs are safe. I have a suspicion that in general, many scientists are far from open-minded.

Nothing shames the providers of medicine—the political and medical establishment. They are quite prepared to extemporise, prevaricate and disbelieve for the purpose of self interest and political expediency. In the meantime, patients have their lives destroyed without redress. It is an intolerable situation and it must change. There is a belief in government and amongst officials and prescribers, that an iatrogenic addict is still an addict and therefore in some way deserving of his situation. The defenders of the status quo demonstrate a raw and breathtaking ability to ignore the ethical implications of the word iatrogenic. There is a hidden battle going on at the moment in medicine, with drug producers, medicine regulators and government on the one hand and disenfranchised and abused patients on the other. The only real question is—how many patients will suffer and die before establishment self interest is generally seen for what it is, and something better is demanded of right. Where else but in mind drug medicine would it be deemed acceptable to kill and maim with impunity—not through human error but through the maintenance of entrenched pharmaceutical, medical and political interests?

In any bureaucratic organisation there will be elements of professionalism, amateurism, ignorance and indifference. The proportions of the mix have no bearing on the continuing existence of the bureaucracy, which if it has political acceptance and approval, will maintain its negative impact on lives. For the organisation, continued existence is the main aim. For the outsider, the focus is on the effect on individuals of the amateurism, indifference and ignorance. Nowhere is this reality more observable than in the damage done to many thousands of lives by psychopharmacology, promoted by establishment medicine as incontrovertibly backed by scientific evidence. The message of gold standard drugs is formulated by the producers of the drugs and accepted by unquestioning politicians, who provide the frontline defence against reality. Attempts by those on the receiving end of benzodiazepines to inform this process, have met over the decades, with blind non-logic and determined resistance from the self-interest of medicine providers, government and its bureaucracies.

According to Plato, Socrates was condemned to death because he did not believe in the gods recognised by the state. Today these gods have been replaced by bureaucrats and experts. Having an expert on tap to deny or minimise the world described by those outside a power system such as medicine, is extremely handy for the modern politician. The existence of bureaucracies, which prevent access to those who could initiate change if they chose to, is even handier.

Benzodiazepines and other psychotropic drugs routinely kill and maim individuals and take away their humanity and freedom because of the existence in the public mind of three enduring myths:

1. That doctors will always act as guardians from harm and act in the patient interest.
2. That drug regulators will protect prescribers and the public from the impact of harmful drugs.
3. That pharmaceutical companies use rigorous and honest science in producing drugs and make marketing subservient to the needs of patients—that the prime reason for their existence is the benefit of humanity.

None of these things is ultimately true, but it suits medicine, its power establishment and most significantly government, to declare their belief in these things and perpetuate their reality. For the UK government and its doctors, psychiatric labelling and the prescription of benzodiazepines has been free at the point of delivery, but has left thousands of individuals far from free. The cost to the existing and future health of patients, their life chances and relationships, has been enormous and often irreversible.

Regulators and prescribers think a great deal about the concept of risk/benefit, but on examination it is a concept which would fit more easily into the world of accountancy. The word 'risk' specifically applies to the patient as it does to the investor, and that is how the providers of medicine like it to be. The patient takes the risk, often without warnings and limited information, owns the risk and is responsible for the consequences of the risk. Substitute the word harm for 'benefit' and you can see how it changes the picture. The word 'harm' points unerringly to the medicine and the providers and prescribers of it. No one who licenses, or who prescribes psychotropic drugs seems willing to understand that both in essence and practice, they are not medicines but controlled substances used as medicines.

The harm done by psychotropic medicine in general has a lot to do with the historical desire of doctors to achieve power through the control of drugs, beginning with their 19th Century victory in gaining control of opium. Dominance, once achieved has necessarily led to a need to maintain that control. The message has been perpetuated that these drugs, uncontrolled in individual hands, are safe in theirs—but that is predicated on the drugs being safe in the first place and on their ability to closely monitor patients for observable signs of side-effects. All mind altering drugs have over time been proved to be unsafe, and enthusiastic and uncontrolled prescribing has often been substituted for close patient monitoring. Drug companies have seen this desire in medicine for control and have exploited it in a great many ways. It has been the exploitation of a medical mindset.

How expert are prescribers?

> "The most serious problems [in medicine] have arisen not because doctors didn't know enough—but because so many behaved as if they did."
> "The fact that doctors want to help and heal patients does not necessarily mean that the power of medicine will be used well...Medicine is still a long way from being as dedicated as government, drug companies and the medical profession would have everyone believe."
> "The present system suits the providers quite well. There is a high degree of unity and inter-dependence between them—notably because of the investment each has in perpetuating the view that the benefits of medicines are overwhelming. Consumers have traditionally been kept at a distance from this tight alliance of government, industry and the mainstream medical profession."
> Charles Medawar, 'Power and Dependence', 1992

> "In my view there's a conspiracy of silence...I believe the problem [benzodiazepine addiction] exists because at a fundamental level, it is too huge and too horrific for people to cope with and grasp the enormity of."
> Phil Woolas MP, 2003

In late 2003 on the terrace of the House of Commons, Phil Woolas MP, a Labour government whip, later Deputy Leader of the House and in 2007 a local government minister, spoke at a meeting to publicise the tabling of a Commons Early Day motion which sought recognition of the damage of benzodiazepine addiction. He explored the question of the scale of damage with his audience. He said:

> "Statistics show that something in the order of 1.2 million people in this country are still in receipt of repeat prescriptions of benzodiazepines, some 20 or 30 years after the danger of that repeat prescription became well known."

Who was maintaining this level of addiction? Obviously the people handing out the pills were doctors, many of whom had carried on traditional prescribing practices long after the negative impact of benzodiazepines should have been known to them, not least through guidance from the Committee on Safety of Medicines, stating quite clearly that prescribing should be focused and for a very short time. The fact that government, regulators, local health employers and the General Medical Council saw it as no business of theirs after that, to either monitor medical behaviour or to control it, was crucially important for the continuation of the damage. But the primary responsibility has to be held by doctors whose defence of what they did is examined later. Campaigner Barry Haslam, himself a victim of a decade long prescribed addiction to Ativan (lorazepam), has fought tenaciously over the years for recognition of the widespread scandal. At the House of Commons meeting, he said something which many patients know to be entirely true:

> "For me, Government Ministers are cowards. If they had gone through one-hundredth of what I've gone through then they would have done something about this long ago. Why have GPs and psychiatrists been allowed to ride roughshod over the advice of people more qualified to judge the drugs than they are? And why have the Government looked the other way? Why have they allowed so many people to get addicted to a legal drug and not put any money into services to help people?"

These questions have been asked by the victims of medical prescribing for decades, and the saddest fact is that they are still being asked, without receiving intelligent answers. Benzodiazepine tranquillisers and hypnotics may provide relief from worry, care, and sleeplessness in the short-term but they are potentially devastating in the longer term. Patients and families live in despair in a situation for which no one will take responsibility and no one within the medical profession or in government is prepared to confront in any direct and meaningful way. The benzodiazepine-affected read critiques from politicians on the rise of the 'compensation culture' and they are confronted with adverts on television telling anyone who has experienced an accident which was not their fault, that they deserve and are entitled to compensation because of it. No one in medicine, or in government, or the manufacturers, has ever compensated anyone, or tried to make their lives easier. It is not actually possible to recompense with money those whose health has been shattered and whose lives have been shortened or lost. But money helps to make coping with the results easier.

> "When doctors err, and the patient dies, doctors don't pay the price for their miscalculation, or poor judgement, or ignorance

> about the adverse effects of many of the drugs they prescribe."
> Alliance for Human Research Protection, 2005

On 26 April 2007, the BBC ran a story under the heading, 'Health gap widest in retirement'. As reported in the British Medical Journal, researchers at University College London followed more than 10,000 British civil servants aged 35 to 55, over a period of twenty years. The research found that a lifetime on a low wage physically ages a person eight years earlier than high earners. Thousands of benzodiazepine victims lost their jobs and many were forced into a hidden, but real and desperate poverty, through the actions of their doctors. Substitute even lower level sickness benefits for low wage and what this research is saying is that doctors have not only inflicted ongoing symptoms but have effectively shortened the functioning lives of large numbers of their patients.

The research gave as an example the fact that the average physical health of a seventy year old high earner was similar to the physical health of a low earner around eight years younger. For the tranquilliser addicted, retirement effectively begins at the time of addiction. What is true is that not only do the addicted face the adverse health effects of the drugs as cited in other chapters in this book, but they also face a further impact because of medically-inflicted poverty. This often begins well before retirement age and not infrequently continues thereafter.

The lead researcher suggested a number of factors could explain the differences found, including lifestyle habits and income. The addicted, living on low levels of state benefit, with restricted abilities regarding food, clothing and lifestyle, encounter all the negative effects of these factors. Help the Aged commented:

> "We need to improve older people's lives and make sure they have a good income in retirement, but also ensure they have good access to improve their health—a good diet and social activities."

Many benzodiazepine dependent people were unable to leave their houses, or even a room for years. Not only were social activities therefore impossible, but their incomes gave them no choices in the primary areas of living. Access to healthcare they may have had, but it was that healthcare system which had caused their downfall. There is no antidote to the effects on health of benzodiazepines but had government ever taken the situation seriously, they could at least have ensured that an adequate income was provided for victims. This Gordian knot, made through uncontrolled medical prescribing, is a tangle that no one sees as their responsibility to cut.

Nearly half a century ago, Librium, Valium and Mogadon were the new wonder pills and for much of the time afterwards drug companies fed this message to doctors. Today the suffering they have inflicted still continues with patients long-addicted, those who have fought free and those who are still being addicted. As government and doctors wash their hands and avoid responsibility, there is no acknowledgement and no support.

The medical profession as a group now likes to believe that tranquillisers are a distant problem of the past and may not have been all that serious anyway—addiction can be dealt with and the problem does not go much further than that. Benzodiazepine drugs are widely considered to belong to a previous generation, replaced in the treatment of insomnia and all manner of modern anxieties by more sophisticated drugs. The problem with that belief is that it is entirely wrong. The situation in the past was serious—almost beyond description, but the unaddressed consequences are still there. The newer drugs which the more up to date experts in the surgeries are now prescribing are Z drugs such as Zaleplon and Zopiclone and the new staunchly defended SSRIs. Both are addictive, and Z drugs in particular have much the same side-effects as benzodiazepines.

But doctors have not given up on benzodiazepines. There are in 2007 around 12 million benzodiazepine prescriptions a year, the slack being taken up by four million Z drug prescriptions and 31 million antidepressant prescriptions. The antidepressant situation is itself odd, since the present official medical creed is that the SSRI predecessors, such as tricyclics and MAOIs, were drugs with greater side-effects, yet they are still prescribed in almost equal measure.

The Department of Health has no accurate figures indicating how many patients are receiving repeat prescriptions of benzodiazepines, or for how long they take them. Professor Heather Ashton, who ran a withdrawal clinic for more than a decade, believes there are at the moment, half a million people in the UK who have been taking benzodiazepines for several years.

The Home Office has figures, for the number of deaths in England and Wales in which drug poisoning is included in coroners' reports. Between 1997 and 2000, cocaine was included in 273 reports, while diazepam and temazepam—only two of the 17 available for prescription—were included in 795. Benzodiazepines however are in drug category C in the Home Office list while cocaine is Class A. Medical over-prescribing has now led to an inexorable rise in the use of benzodiazepines on the street and hence their involvement in the deaths of illegal users.

The statistics of the medically dependent and the numbers of illegal users are significant because it is a problem inflicted by doctors in a national health service. Prescribed addiction is so common that surreally, it is ignored in the formulation of drug policies and the funding of withdrawal treatment. This is largely due to the near-the-throne drug advisers who hide the problem and obfuscate its reality, and the desire of government to keep the lid on a can of worms for which they are ultimately responsible. For government the preservation of the NHS image and the protection of a scarce medical resource—the number of doctors, is a primary motivation. Tranquilliser dependence is fortunately an addiction where victims largely suffer in silence, kept quiet by their repeat prescriptions from doctors' surgeries.

Most experiences of involuntary addiction follow a common theme of suffering during prescription, and suffering afterwards. Benzodiazepines are often the 'damned when you take them', 'damned when you stop' drugs. Those who have become aware of this cannot understand why such an aggressive drug is still in the uncontrolled hands of doctors.

What is the nature of the science which was sold to doctors and on which they based their expertise?

In the late fifties Dr Alec Jenner was working at the United Hospital in Sheffield. He had read of a Swiss circus trainer who had a drug which calmed lions and tigers. In the noblest scientific traditions of medicine, he asked himself whether such a drug might do something positive for the human population.

Jenner contacted Roche, whose scientific researcher, Leo Sternbach, had almost accidentally discovered the chemical compound which became Librium in 1959 and later Valium and Mogadon. Roche of course were highly delighted that an independent researcher had voluntarily asked to try out something which they had plans to sell to doctors as a safe alternative to barbiturates. They were more than happy to accept his offer to do studies which would aid future marketing.

Before Jenner, the benefit message was merely based on a series of impressions and the possibility of serious long-term effects had never been subjected to rigorous scientific examination. Jenner has admitted to nothing much more than being naive when carrying out what he thinks were the first double blind trials. Volunteers were given two bottles A and B, and were told what might be in them without saying which bottle contained what. In his benzodiazepine trials, the bottles contained either a barbiturate, a benzodiazepine compound, or a placebo. Jenner has said he believes the number of subjects studied was around 200. He apparently does not seem to have considered at the time that the small population studies, carried out over limited time on drugs which were later taken by millions—many over years and decades, were not conclusively describing benefit.

Jenner had never seen drug addicts and seemed to believe that addiction potential was something outside his scientific remit—although he subsequently said that it seemed rather mad that he had not considered it.

Many subsequently addicted patients have a lot more than that to say. But the inadequate trials were gratefully received by Roche and added what they claimed was independent scientific underpinning of their message to doctors.

There were other studies carried out at the same time, but they did not consider the possibility of addiction either. This allowed Roche's researchers in New Jersey, to issue a report in 1961 emphasising the few side-effects of the newly discovered chemical, though it is salutary that the message of limited, mild side-effects was based on a study of only seven subjects. There had been nine patients but the results of two of them were not included because side-effects had forced them to drop out. On average patients took Valium for three months.

This was the standard of the science which drug regulators in the UK accepted as demonstrating much benefit and little risk attached to the drug Valium, launched in the UK in 1963. Roche and the other manufacturers of subsequent copycat drugs have never investigated long-term effects and regulators have never required them to. The long-term studies have been done by patients and their families but the results of that experience is largely discounted and marginalised. Those studies after all were not scientific, merely the reflection of practical experience. Manufacturers on the other hand, with a message not backed by science but by marketing, were allowed to give the impression to doctors that here was a whole new world of beneficial drugs, almost entirely free of side-effects.

> "The entire impression was given to doctors deliberately that a real revolution had occurred and it was time to change their prescribing habits and use these drugs for the benefit, as you might say, of mankind."
> Professor Graham Dukes, WHO Adviser, 2001

Benzodiazepine manufacturers produced wondrous advertising images so that doctors could see for themselves how beneficial the drugs were. They fought any attempts at control, both in the UK and the US and won. In 1979 in the US, Roche executives, like the tobacco barons, faced a special Senate sub-committee hearing convened to examine the serious question of growing benzodiazepine dependence and bamboozled it. As Charles Medawar has said in his book 'Power and Dependence':

> "The defence of Valium and other benzodiazepines was orchestrated and cast by Roche to an extent which doctors could not have appreciated."

This should not of course imply that because the message coming from regulators and pharmaceutical companies was one of wonder, that doctors should be absolved from blame. The history described, merely serves to illustrate how expert doctors really were, when they addicted unsuspecting patients in their tens of thousands to one of the world's most addictive substances. By 1979 when the world consumption of benzodiazepines was estimated at 3 billion prescriptions, much had been written about problems with the drugs but UK doctors still kept on prescribing, as though in a bubble, isolated from rational science and the stories coming from patients.

By 1966, the year of the Rolling Stones' song, 'Mother's Little Helper', Roche had become the world's largest pharmaceutical company. Seeing this success the other large pharmaceutical companies were inspired to jump on the bandwagon and produce their own benzodiazepines. Wyeth grew rich on Ativan and Upjohn produced Xanax. It might be of interest to note that between the wars, Roche had been involved in illegal drug running and had been prosecuted several times. In 1927 the Chairman of the British delegation to the Opium Advisory Committee of the League of Nations asserted that he had:

> "...no doubt whatever that Hoffmann-La Roche and Company was not a firm to which a licence to deal with drugs should be given."

In the hallowed tradition of most medical scientists, Jenner was sceptical about the evidence of harm—it takes a lot of evidence to convince a scientist when his claim to fame is invested in the opposite message. Jenner was a member of the Committee on Safety of Medicines, and probably represents an example of why it takes regulators so long to produce guidelines aimed at the protection of patients.

This quote from Jenner illustrates, more than anything, the divide between human pharmacological science and human lives:

> "I feel naive but not guilty. What seemed so good about the benzodiazepines **when I was playing with them** was that it seemed like we really did have a drug that didn't have many problems. But in retrospect it's difficult to put a spanner into a wristwatch and expect that it won't do any harm." [My emphasis]

Retrospection is something scientists may have an opportunity to indulge, but patients fed the results of the drugs they underwrote, are often not given that opportunity.

In July 2006, Professor Sir Mike Rawlins, Professor of Pharmacology at Newcastle University, who is also chairman of the National Institute for Health and Clinical Excellence, (NICE) said:

> "A great deal of mis-prescribing is because of a lack of knowledge. About 80% of adverse drug reactions are avoidable...Deaths due to adverse drug reactions have risen by over 500% since the early 1990s and are now estimated to cost the NHS £500m a year."

Professor Jeffrey Aronson, from Oxford, then the new president-elect of the British Pharmacological Society, said:

> "I think that a lot of this is actually preventable..."

But is it excusable? When injury should be avoidable why is it not avoided? Both men were confirming the reality of the extent of medical prescribing expertise. Benzodiazepine patients have died and been harmed through the use of drugs which were licensed without the backing of rigorous science and which were poorly regulated. But ultimately it is because doctors, in acceptance of this sea of sand, still believed in their expertise.

In December 1998, campaigner Sue Bibby was interviewed on Talk Radio and described the result of the non-expertise of psychiatrists and GPs. She told the interviewer:

> "...apart from people's physical health going down (although luckily, some people seem to be able to stand up to that), they are described by their families as being "Jekyll and Hyde". Agoraphobia (not being able to go out) is a very, very common symptom which very few people actually have before they're given the drugs—sometimes they might have it, but mostly they don't have it until they've been put on the drugs. This of course makes them [the patients] incapable of doing anything much. They can't go out to the local shops; they can't look after their children properly. They are very distressed by this and feel it's their own fault. Usually they go back to the GP and the GP will say: "Oh you're an anxious personality and that's what's wrong with you," and they usually give them more benzodiazepines or other antidepressant drugs as well."

Clinical judgement is enshrined in medicine, but to have clinical judgement, drugs would have to be realistically researched, honestly promoted, closely monitored after licensing, and all known side-effects communicated as soon as they are observed. Additionally doctors would have to be sufficiently motivated to keep abreast of developments and see it as their responsibility to warn patients in advance. Only one in ten side-effects is ever notified by doctors. They are not overly proficient at noticing the negative potential of licensed drugs. Some may not be very concerned.

Professor Malcolm Lader, writing in the Journal of Substance Abuse Treatment in 1991 on the history of benzodiazepine dependence said:

> "The widespread usage of the benzodiazepines has inevitably led to thousands of people becoming dependent. Patients who have become dependent and have either been able to withdraw or have only done so with great symptomatic distress, justifiably feel aggrieved against their doctors."

This justifiable grievance has in part perhaps something to do with the inability of prescribers to deal with the consequences of their actions. As Professor Lader said on the Discovery Channel programme 'In Pills We Trust' in December 2002:

> "Doctors were not well equipped to deal with this [benzodiazepine withdrawal]. They don't like dealing with chronic drug use or addiction anyway."

Perhaps doctors have never subjected themselves to an analysis of their skills, because they have routinely carried on addicting patients anyway.
In the Sunday Express Magazine in 1999 under the headline, 'More addictive than heroin, yet prescribed to one in four adults. Benzodiazepines can ruin lives...' Robert Kerwin, Professor of Psychopharmacology at the Maudsley Hospital, London described the situation:

> "A lot of people have been damaged by the over-prescribing of benzodiazepines. They get repeat prescriptions—and then they get stuck on them. Symptoms include intense anxiety, panic attacks and sleeplessness. But if a patient got these, doctors just put it down to their disorder and re-prescribed benzodiazepines. What they are being used for is not the original condition—but just preventing the withdrawal syndrome. Users go through life semi-tranquillised in a state of hypnosis. They're still being doled out without much thought."

Professor Heather Ashton confirmed the effect of the drugs:

> "One common feeling among long-term users is that they have spent years in a kind of daze. Many cannot remember their children growing up and this is one of their most bitter regrets. These drugs dampen down everything in the brain so when you come off them you get this rebound state. You're very sensitive to physical stimuli. In some cases this never settles down."

Malcolm Lader describes in his article possible reasons why doctors kept on harming patients. He said:

> "Some older doctors just don't want to change, and they're still giving out repeat prescriptions. Some GPs also deny the drugs' effects, arguing that their patients have addictive personalities. Yet one of the most common benzodiazepines, diazepam (brand name Valium), is also used in patients with sports injuries as a muscle relaxant. We found that people without any psychiatric condition at all have the same withdrawal problem."

But when the expert with a public voice apparently contradicts himself, is there now absolution for the anointed?

> "There is a most substantial body of evidence that confirms the effect of these drugs [benzodiazepines] as broadly deleterious to lucid thought, comprehension, understanding, decision making and judgemental abilities."
> Professor Ian Hindmarch, University of Surrey, **1997**

> "It's true that you can become dependent on benzodiazepines; I think even the most serious critics will say that the percentage of people who use benzodiazepines and become clinically dependent is under 4%, which means that 96% can use these drugs without any dependency or problems whatsoever."
> Professor Ian Hindmarch, University of Surrey, Radio 4,
> **December 2003**

When government turns it face away from reality where can there be exculpation?

> "Tinkering with the legislation is not sufficient. Government has a role and a serious role. Talking about Drugs Tsars [and] Wars on Drugs misses the point. You are dealing with people who are damaged, people who have deep mental pain and therefore you have to find the best practice, persuasion and encouragement."
> Dr Bob Johnson, 'Mother's Little Killers', Channel 4 News,
> January 4 2001

In July 2006 we were told that doctors were to face competence checks to ensure they were fit to practise. Sir Liam Donaldson, the government's

Chief Medical Officer said that patient safety had to be his primary concern and therefore there must be a robust revalidation process. As he said:

> "At present, a senior doctor can go through a thirty year career without undergoing a single assessment of their fitness to practise, whereas an airline pilot, meanwhile, would face over 100 checks over a similar timescale."

Of course the question of whether drugs are being prescribed according to official guidelines should be examined, but when the drugs themselves are inherently dangerous, side-effect information is poorly analysed and restricted, and guidelines are invariably many years late, it is doubtful whether patients will be effectively protected by the type of competence checks proposed. Nevertheless, doctors do not want their world examined too closely. James Johnson, chairman of the doctors' trade union, the British Medical Association, attacked the plans to change the burden of guilt:

> "It seems wrong to be able to take away a doctor's livelihood because of something found on a balance of probability rather than proving something beyond reasonable doubt. It opens the door to miscarriages of justice which will devastate the lives of doctors and their families."

No recognition sadly that doctors have devastated the lives of many thousands through incompetence. Joyce Robins, co-director of Patient Concern asked:

> "Why can't we just implement these desperately needed changes to improve protection of patients?"

On 24th April 2007, the Daily Mail in 'The great depression swindle' cited a study done by Dr Alex Mitchell, a consultant psychiatrist at Leicester General Hospital. It found that 62% of patients diagnosed with depression were not depressed. There had been a gross over-estimation by GPs and psychiatrists of the number of people who are depressed. Under the latest government guidelines, doctors are paid extra to ask patients two simple questions. The answers are supposedly designed to show if you are depressed or not. The two questions are:

- During the past month have you been bothered by feeling down, depressed or hopeless?
- During the past month have you been bothered by having little interest or pleasure in doing things?

Given the acknowledged and the unacknowledged serious side-effects associated with antidepressants, why would a healing profession wish to give drugs to those who are in fact healthy? The questions, approved by the National Institute for Clinical Excellence (NICE) in 2004, are an example of the low degree of forethought and analysis that goes into the diagnosis of mental illness. The tick box culture in medicine has been recently criticised in America and as Professor Ashton commented in April 2007:

> “Most psychiatrists still seem to use the DSM as a bible. Psychiatry still seems to be at the stage of pinning butterflies and beetles into boxes like the Victorian naturalists. It is OK as a start to classification but far too rigid and a bar to progress if adhered to too strictly.”

Once you've ticked enough boxes for symptoms, you receive a diagnosis of depression even though in actual fact you may just be normally sad. And the consequences thereafter are your own responsibility.

There are 250,000 serious adverse reactions to a pharmaceutical drug reported every year in the UK. This is a very conservative estimate, and is based only on reported reactions. A truer figure is believed to be closer to 1,200,000 every year. In the United States, where medicine is even more aggressive, the situation could be affecting up to 13,450,000 people every year. It is a fact, acknowledged even by government, that there is a massive under-reporting of mistakes and injury. Nobody knows how many of the reported blunders end in the death of the patient. Only 1 out of 4 hospitals ‘owns up’ to the patient when something goes wrong; the rest blame it on the disease itself, while just 1 in 25 drug reactions is ever reported. Edward Leigh, Chairman of the Commons Public Accounts committee commenting on the figures has said:

> "These figures would be terrifying enough without our learning that there is undoubtedly substantial under-reporting of serious incidents and deaths. To top it all, the NHS simply has no idea how many people die each year from patient safety incidents."

Hospital staff gave the wrong treatment to the wrong patient on almost 25,000 occasions in 2006, leading to both death and long-term injury according to official figures from the National Patient Safety Agency. There was no analysis of the figures available to show how many patients had died or been seriously harmed but the agency managed to admit that the overall total could be much higher due to many incidents being unreported. The NPSA reported 41,000 medication errors between July 2005 and July 2006, causing 36 deaths. For 2004, the National Audit Office said there had been nearly one million errors, causing 2,000 deaths. The NAO estimated that half of the incidents could have been avoided if staff had learnt from past mistakes. On the face of it there had been a large improvement in the figures for death in 2004, the figures for 2005 and perhaps the figures for 2006 but who would trust such statistics?

Prescribers and hospital staff are not learning from the mistakes, but are merely repeating them year after year. Guidelines are being consistently ignored, and safety recommendations are not being implemented. Patients have nowhere to turn, and it can be extremely difficult to prove a case of medical malpractice when hospitals and doctors constantly deny there has been a problem. The National Patient Safety Agency says it receives thousands of calls a month from people saying they have been victims of a medical accident.

2006 figures from the British Medical Association, the doctors' trade union, said that at least 250,000 people end up in hospital every year because of the damaging side-effects of the medicines they are taking and about 5,000 die. In pursuance of patient protection the Association urged their members to be more vigilant and report any suspected side-effects their patients might experience. But ten years ago, the BMA issued similar guidance to doctors, and it had little effect. The reports of what patients tell doctors to the Medicines and Healthcare products Agency have remained at around 20,000 since the mid 1980s. Various reasons, from having too much to do, to not having a supply of yellow cards to fill in, to lethargy, have been put forward.

In 2004 a study in Liverpool by Dr M Pirmohamed, Professor of Clinical Pharmacology at Liverpool University, and others, said that more than 10,000 people a year may die from the side-effects of medicines prescribed by their doctors and most of those deaths are unnecessary. The question asked by patients is what is a necessary death? Deaths due to adverse drug reactions have risen by over 500% since the early 1990s.

Whatever the true extent of the figures, the reality is that medical expertise is often a myth. But it is a myth that most people want to believe. This is in spite of the fact that even a drug maker has said something illuminating on the subject of drug benefit. In December 2003 Dr Allen Roses, of GlaxoSmithKline, was quoted in a national newspaper as saying more than 90% of drugs only work in 30–50% of people. Of course he could have made a stab at the percentage of people who take drugs which not only do not work for them but actually cause them harm—but he did not.

Perhaps patients would be well advised to heed the words of Dr James Le Fanu in the Daily Telegraph on 8 November 2006:

> "The best of treatments must be the friendly reassurance that, whatever the symptoms, they will pass and there is no need to take pills or potions to relieve them. Or, as wise old Hippocrates put it, "to do nothing is also a good remedy". His aphorism should be inscribed above the door of every surgery, certainly given the response to last week's column, which featured the woman whose general practitioner was trying to persuade her she was "not as well as I thought I was" and treating her for illnesses she did not have...It is difficult to convey the sheer insouciance with which readers describe being told, on the flimsiest of grounds, that they have some potentially serious illness and the need for long-term medication."

Patients die or are seriously harmed because drug companies have carried out biased research, because regulators accept that research as demonstrating safety and because of the lack of ongoing safety monitoring by either. The fourth and crucial element is that **doctors lack sufficient knowledge to prescribe drugs properly.**

Professor (not then Sir) Michael Rawlins, who prior to his role with NICE, became head of the Committee on Safety of Medicines in 1992, had come to much the same conclusion after research he did as far back as 1988. This begs the question, as it always does, about who is responsible for initiating change and who is in charge of making sure the change is effective and timely. Dr Andrew Herxheimer as Consultant Pharmacologist at Charing Cross Hospital in London, agreed with the research but pointed out something which is vitally important, and that is that any figures on hospital fatality or harm due to drugs are unlikely to be accurate because hospital admissions of drug-damaged patients take no account of those who remain at home under the care of a GP.

This issue of drug safety should have been effectively addressed with benzodiazepines decades ago but it never has been, and as a result, an underclass of drug survivors has been created, struggling through their lives with poor health and no economic security. In the meantime, doctors have maintained their right to expertise in prescribing.

There is no doubt that most doctors regard themselves as unique, occupying a special niche in society and owed regard above and beyond the regard owed to ordinary mortals. In June 2005, the BBC aired a programme called 'Real Story' on the subject of medical addictions to alcohol and drugs. The programme claimed that one in fifteen doctors is addicted to either drugs or drink. Figures were obtained by using the Freedom of Information Act and showed that in the past decade 750 clinical and medical staff had been formally disciplined for offences involving alcohol or drugs at work. The BBC survey was based on replies from one in three hospital trusts in the UK. A patient from Folkestone told Real Story that she had been seen by a doctor who had come in straight from riding, paralytic, all over the place and slurring, but according to the logic of medicine, the person most in need of deserving protection and help here was the doctor.

The British Medical Association, rather than recoiling in horror at this threat to the safety of patients preferred to point out that the scale of the problem is no worse than for the general population, as though this view (even if it is true) somehow absolves the profession from responsibility. Dr Vivienne Nathanson, the BMA's head of science and ethics said:

> "...doctors work in very stressful environments in a culture where it is difficult to seek help. There are some services already available to doctors such as the BMA's counselling service and its advisory unit, Doctors for Doctors, but the government could do more by investing in specially designed services that will meet the distinct needs of doctors."

On the other hand, what Dr Nathanson seems to be unaware of is the fact that those the profession have turned into drug addicts through their prescribing of benzodiazepines, do not find any of their needs met by government or the medical profession either. Many benzodiazepine addicts have their lives turned into a global experience of stress, unable to work, without choices, personal pensions, normal relationships or health.

How doctors defend their actions

> "How do you deal with something unpleasant? The commonest way is not to think about it. That, I suspect, is why medicine has paid so little attention to the harm it may cause—despite the ancient instruction "first, do no harm"...every intervention by a doctor, even a throwaway comment or a test "just to be sure," carries the potential for harm, whereas many of those interventions have no possibility of bringing benefit...
> Very few people attend a doctor thinking that they may come out worse than when they went in. But many do."
> Richard Smith, Editor, British Medical Journal, July 2004

In essence, doctors are never required to explain their actions when it finally becomes acceptable to recognise that a particular drug has inflicted harm. The nature of the defence they do provide is thin and has very little to do with health protection. Here is a typical example of how their trade union sees the issue of benzodiazepine dependence:

> “Some people have been on the drugs for many years and it is very difficult to get them off because they are very addictive. We can nibble away at the problem—but it is a very time intensive thing to have to do.”
> Dr Peter Fellowes, Chairman BMA Prescribing Committee, March 2004

Is there any recognition in this statement that it was doctors who created what is euphemistically termed ‘the problem’? The description ‘very addictive’ is there, but it took very many years before that admission appeared. And then we have the great excuse, and here is the line of thought—Yes, benzodiazepines are very addictive and we prescribed them to produce the addiction, but we will not talk about that. What we will say, after reducing the numbers of addicted from tens of thousands to ‘some’, is that doing anything about it is beyond us because we do not have the time. Therefore it must surely be somebody else’s responsibility and if that responsibility remains unfilled, we cannot be blamed for that.

Go back three years and we have another statement, this time from the professional body of those responsible for the majority of the addiction. The distorted grammar is as it was spoken:

> “I think it should be a significant priority for this country. It's potentially a million people who are on drugs which only maybe is a tiny percentage of them need to be on, and that is not good for this country. It's also a waste of resource. We are ploughing money into these drugs and into support services for patients for a situation that we **may** have created ourselves.” [My emphasis]
> Dr Jim Kennedy, (Royal College of General Practitioners)
> ‘The Tranquilliser Trap’, BBC 2001

What is being said here? Maybe a million people are affected by the prescribed addiction, somewhat above the BMA estimate of ‘some’, in 2004. No expression of regret or shame. There is a recognition that here is something that requires the action of those with the power to address it, but no real emphasis on the fact that it is a medically-induced epidemic. The impression is given that the ‘problem’ is being addressed and it is very costly to do it. Support services are specifically mentioned as being part of the great expense but what if these support services exist only in the mind of Jim Kennedy? What if the cost of the drugs is actually a drop in the ocean compared with the cost if government recognised the disabled, those unable to work, those forced into the dark corners of society by medicine? In the Oldham Chronicle on 14 May 2007, Phil Woolas MP told the reporter:

> "We must ask why is Oldham, the only Primary Care Trust in the country which pays for the service [Oldham Withdrawal Project]. And officials must come up from the Department of Health to study Oldham's model and see if it can be replicated across the country."

In January 2004, Sir Liam Donaldson, the government's Chief Medical Officer wrote in Update 37, a communication to all doctors:

> "General Practitioners in England wrote 12.7 million prescriptions at a cost of £20.9 million in 2002."

In 1999 Charles Medawar of Social Audit on the BBC programme 'Face the Facts' said:

> "The cost to the NHS of benzodiazepine dependence is not high. The fact is that you can maintain somebody on a prescription of benzodiazepines for 'pence per month'."

You have to ask why it is that the Royal College of General Practitioners maintains that the country is ploughing money into support services for medically dependent patients and into the cost of the drugs themselves. Even the Chief Medical Officer is saying that in 2002 the drugs cost a mere £21 million, though presumably he was making an effort to impress doctors with that figure. Phil Woolas and benzodiazepine campaigners know that support services, outside Oldham in the North of England do not exist.

Jim Kennedy refers to a waste of resource. He is referring to the cost to the NHS—but what about the human cost? There are dead people, people incredibly injured by benzodiazepines, people addicted many years ago, who because there was no help and no information, were never given the chance to withdraw and as a consequence could not work, forced to live a life of ever increasing distress. If a life can be seen as a completed jigsaw then for large numbers of people, over the years of their medical addiction, they have—usually without comprehension, watched as the pieces were being gradually disassembled.

Kennedy also said on the same BBC programme in 2001:

> "There is still a significant continuing problem with benzodiazepines in this country. We would have liked if it was solved 20 years ago, but it still exists. We continue to work as a College with prescribing groups around the country to try and continue to raise awareness of this issue and reduce the prescribing of these drugs to appropriate use, but it is a very long struggle."

It is unfortunate that nobody on the programme asked him why preventing death, health damage and addiction, was a struggle that had taken twenty years and was still ongoing. In any other sphere of life, such a situation would not be tolerated. There is a heavy price to be paid by some for the general belief in the expertise, humanity and effectiveness of doctors.

The Royal College of GPs believes the reasons long-term use continues are varied—patients choose to stay on the drugs, people ask for them, time and resources for careful withdrawal are not available, or due to length of use, withdrawal must be undertaken gradually, with doses being reduced marginally over a period of months. This defence against logic and any sense of responsibility is widely used in medicine. When analysed, it always seems to boil down to a deflection of even mild criticism in the direction of the patient and when this is deemed to be insufficient, towards 'them', presumably meaning government and local health authorities. Bemusingly, government and local health employers, when approached, deflect pleas for action in the direction of those doing the prescribing. This statement from Dr John McCormack, General Medical Council, on BBC 'Face the Facts', in March 1999 is an illustration of the deflection towards 'them':

> "This is a worldwide problem [benzodiazepine dependence] and I think one of the big factors is they're cheap. GPs are now under a great deal of pressure to prescribe inexpensive drugs. Now, a thousand 2mg Valium tablets...diazepam tablets ...cost around £3 which is not very much. If you are prescribed 60 and you pay the six quid prescription fee, the government makes a nice little profit out of you."

Most of these arguments apply to all psychotropic drugs, but were historically formulated to deal with the benzodiazepine question. The Times on 14 May 2007 declared that Britain was becoming a Prozac nation. It described how in 2006 UK doctors had written out just over 31 million prescriptions for antidepressants. This was a big increase on previous years, in the face of widespread evidence of possible addiction and severe and sometimes fatal side-effects. The story was almost a re-run of the benzodiazepine story—30.9 million benzodiazepine prescriptions in 1979: 31 million antidepressant prescriptions in 2006.

Doctors have obviously failed to adopt scepticism about new wonder pills and significantly, many keep on prescribing wonder pills after the clouds have formed. Half of the 31 million figure for antidepressants was made up of tricyclics, which have been known for a long time to be far less than a wonder treatment. Like amateurs, not experts, they have picked up on the criticism in recent years of the latest wonder drugs SSRIs and have gravitated back to drugs which came before. Or perhaps some have not progressed beyond the prescription of the older drugs which they believe work for them, just as some have never wavered from the belief that benzodiazepines are not as black as they are painted.

As usual, the figures on how many people are taking drugs for depression on a long-term basis are a little fuzzy, just as even today there is no precision about benzodiazepine figures. There is informed criticism of the antidepressant prescribing made by some, just as there was over the benzodiazepine decades—until the media became tired and convinced itself that there was no longer a problem. Paul Farmer, Chief Executive of the mental health charity MIND from May 2006 onwards, said:

> "Doctors are guilty of a knee-jerk reaction in prescribing pills, which are commonly long-term prescriptions and have well-known issues with side-effects. The mindset of GPs will have to change so that they consider counselling and other forms of therapy as a frontline treatment."

Doctors do have a case in saying that counselling is patchy and often not available, in spite of government assurances that it exists. But they do not have a case in believing that therefore, if millions appear in the surgery believing themselves to be depressed, that they then have no alternative but to supply potentially hazardous drugs, when they know full well that they do not have the time to provide any safe degree of monitoring.

A family doctor in Reading in 2007 expressed the caring medical view when he said that patients increasingly expected to be given medication rather than other therapies:

> "Antidepressants seem to have lost the stigma they once had and now most patients seem to want to take them."

What kind of health protection is this? What kind of expertise is being shown? Because drugs have lost their stigma, presumably because the patients badgering doctors are completely unaware of what might happen to them, doctors must fulfil that ignorant need?

Dr Terry Lynch, based in Limerick is known to have concerns about the over-reliance of his profession on medications to treat the problem of mental distress and he has explored the operation of the defence of its actions. In the Sunday Tribune, March 2 2003, he referred back to the benzodiazepine situation:

> "It's now 15 years since the Committee on Safety of Medicines gave its advice about prescribing benzodiazepines, and unfortunately the truth seems to be that they weren't followed."

Then he homed in on the real causes of patient addiction and prescribed drug harm:

> "The problem was created by prescribing, and a considerable part of the problem was created by not paying sufficient attention to what patients were telling us. Historically, we have a problem recognising the addiction potential of medications and acting swiftly on the information—I mean, we had similar problems in the past with barbiturates and amphetamines, more recently with benzodiazepines, and I personally believe that in the future we will have a similar problem with the antidepressants which are so enthusiastically prescribed at the moment."

Following the views of Charles Medawar, Professor Heather Ashton and others, he went on to say:

> "Twenty years ago, benzodiazepines were held as 'wonder drugs', so there is an eerie repetitiveness about this. Each drug that comes along gives doctors a new 'hope' to believe in and to prescribe, and prescribing is second nature to doctors, that is how they are trained. But many of them have a very basic understanding of anxiety and distress and what patients are going through, what is causing their pain."

He recognises the responsibilities of patients to avoid pressurising doctors but at the same time he also recognises that the medical profession inflates this reality, as a means to shifting complete responsibility from themselves as prescribers to those who take the prescriptions, thereby gaining absolution. Mostly he believes the pressure to take drugs comes from the doctor.

Lynch does not accept, as does the British Medical Association and the Royal College of GPs that the profession can hide behind statements that the time is not there to do anything beyond prescribe, or that alternative resources are limited. As he points out, and it is undoubtedly true, no one hears much about doctors pushing for increased counselling services as an alternative to drugs. But most significantly and unusually for a doctor, he has pointed to the crucial need for an effective external apparatus for the independent monitoring and surveillance of the medical profession.

The medical profession as a whole prefers to talk about other things than its responsibilities to improve and protect the health of patients. Indeed in May 2007, the profession launched an attack in what it regards as a crucial area of healthcare—patients are wasting prescription medicines by not completing the course of treatment. Patients were even having the temerity to take their health into their own hands. Amazingly one in five doctors even said patients should be financially penalised for not completing a treatment. They have a point of course, but on the other hand drugs which many patients might well have benefited from wasting include such wonders as the SSRIs, benzodiazepines, Vioxx, Celebrex, Ritalin and antipsychotics. All of these drugs were recommended by doctors as beneficial for various conditions, all of these drugs have killed and maimed enormous numbers of trusting patients. In the five years it was available, Vioxx has been estimated to have killed 60,000 people worldwide. How Vioxx came to be in the hands of British doctors is typical of a large number of drugs. Professor Michael Langman (a member of the Committee on Safety of Medicines, the UK drugs watchdog) with links to Merck which had supported his research became the champion of Vioxx. In 1999, nine days after he sat with the Merck delegation in the US to consider the licence application, the CSM approved the drug for UK use. The first heart attack reports in Britain came within nine months of the product launch. After five years of intense marketing, including an estimated $160 million campaign in Britain in 2001, Merck acknowledged its own and independent findings and withdrew the drug in 2004. But then, as Professor Langman said in August 2005:

> "I don't think I've done anything other than express what I regarded as an honest opinion."

Perhaps what Professor Robin Murray of the Institute of Psychiatry at Kings College, London said in 2004, has relevance here:

> "Academics, particularly academic pharmacologists, have somehow begun to believe that it is acceptable to present company data as if they were a hired gun."

And something which both public and doctors should be aware of is the danger of a blind belief in medical benefit which was nicely encapsulated by biologist Professor, Lord Robert Winston in 2006:

> "Science and religion are both about uncertainty—it's when they become certain that they become dangerous."

Most doctors do not seem to feel the need to become aware of the reality expressed by Professor Bruno Stricker, in the British Medical Journal in 2004. If doctors, rather than hailing each new wonder drug as it came along, would exercise caution, they would do far less damage and there would be far less need to defend it:

“...most experts will agree that the widespread marketing of a new drug is in fact a large experiment on a population. This is especially the case when it concerns a novel molecular entity with potentially a new set of clinical experiences...”

Medicine is a caring profession?

“A clinical psychiatrist and countless GPs have written that prescription [Citalopram] out for me. And never, not once, has anyone taken the time to say "think long and hard, it could be hell when you stop.""
Holly Finch,The Guardian, January 30 2007

“It seems that the more people are exposed to doctors and contemporary healthcare, including the rhetoric of preventative care, the sicker they feel.”
Dr Iona Heath GP, British Medical Journal, April 2005

Doctors apparently do not seem to appreciate that they have any role to play in protecting patients from themselves or drug company spin when it comes to prescribing drugs available on prescription only. At the same time however, there is a never-ending stream of medical advice in the media, warning the public against the dangers of a bewildering variety of things such as caffeine, red meat, alcohol, sunbathing, vitamins, television, and internet connections.

That unreality exists in the minds of medics is illustrated by their dogged and never-ending defence against any accusations that they are routinely overly influenced by pharmaceutical marketing techniques. A report in 2006 by Consumers International, said that doctors were accepting kickbacks, gifts, free samples and consulting agreements in exchange for prescribing or promoting drugs. It said that such inducements accounted for a substantial part of the £33 billion spent on global product promotion by the industry each year. In February 2006, it was discovered that a senior manager at Abbott Laboratories, had taken a hospital doctor to a lap dancing club. Senior hospital consultants were provided with Wimbledon tickets and more than sixty doctors were taken to a greyhound race meeting in Manchester. Commenting on this kind of medical behaviour, Dr Raymond MacAllister, Senior Lecturer in Pharmacology, University of London said in October 2004:

“The profession is under a mass delusion...if the general public knew what was going on, they would be astonished.”

It is something to do with what Professor Edwin Gale, University of Bristol described in the same Guardian article:

> "Doctors are so incredibly gullible because they suspect themselves of the highest motives."

But none of the doctors involved, in their own estimation, would have been influenced by the Pharma freebies and no doctor was disciplined in consequence. The General Medical Council has outlined proposals to restrict this generosity from the makers of drugs, but drug companies are nothing if not resourceful.

In May 2007 four drug companies, Johnson & Johnson, Pfizer, Novartis and Procter & Gamble proposed the launch of a television station to tell the public about their drugs. Intense lobbying is taking place across Europe to bring an end to restrictions on direct advertising to patients. Pharma TV is planned to be a dedicated interactive digital channel funded by the industry with at its heart, information designed to sell drug company medicines directly to the punters. This, if it happens, will mean that the patient will become the consumer rather than the doctor and in that scenario, taking doctors on jaunts will no longer be necessary.

Every survey ever taken points to large public satisfaction with doctors. Why this is has probably much to do with the questions asked, enduring public myths, a lack of personal experience of harm, and an ignorance of pharmaceutical influence. Nevertheless there is dissatisfaction. In 2005, a record number of complaints were made about doctors to the General Medical Council. The number of complaints made to the GMC is still miniscule at 4,980 and there are reasons for that, the most important being a lack of public knowledge regarding the GMC complaints procedure. Many more people contact patients' bodies with complaints.

At a time when hospital wards are closing and GP hours and services are being cut, the salaries of doctors have risen sharply. In the year 2005–6 GPs' average earnings rose to £118,000. At the same time as this was happening it was being discovered that in elderly care homes, thousands were being drugged unnecessarily. More than 22,000 elderly people in nursing homes are being given powerful sedatives for no medical reason. This discovery has been spear-headed by the Liberal Democrat Party which has consistently campaigned on the subject. In their report 'Keep Taking the Medicine' they say that the prescription of powerful anti-psychotics and tranquillisers is increasing year after year. There is clear evidence that care homes are turning to chemical cocktails to make residents easier to manage. The response of the National Care Homes Association was to say, without any sense of irony, that if it was true that the drugs were being prescribed for no clinical reason, merely to make the life of care home staff easier, then it was doctors who needed to be called to account. This has often been said by patients but without success. Given the state of UK law and the lack of action by medical bodies, employers and government, it is not surprising.

In January 2007, we were told that government had plans to offer GPs even more money to start working in the evenings and weekends again. This was three years after the negotiation of a new contract following which the vast majority of GPs stopped out-of-hours work. Ministers are in a quandary after a major patient survey showed growing dissatisfaction with the new service which meant that GPs were no longer responsible for patients in out of office hours. Government is therefore preparing to use the historically effective method of employing financial bribes to encourage GPs to change their working patterns once again.

When the NHS was created, Health Secretary Bevan, to the detriment of future healthcare practices and control, left GPs as small businesses. As a consequence of the recent power-based negotiations by the BMA, most GPs now work forty-four hours a week. It is often difficult to see a doctor, not least because most surgeries are closed in the evenings and also at weekends. Suitable and convenient appointments can be hard to obtain, but the criticism of the new situation is strangely not aimed at doctors who are still regarded as paragons of virtue, imbued with a nobility which in reality is long gone—if it ever generally existed.

GPs used to keep 40% of NHS taxpayers' money for themselves, but in 2006 that has crept up to 45%. The new GP contract ensures that the small businesses have a guaranteed income, with no limits on profit and no competition. In spite of this there is no comeback against failing GPs. As the NHS negotiators have said, only the very worst have their contracts ended. The very worst probably do not include those who give no help to addicted patients and who continue to addict them.

In negotiations over pay for 2007, the GPs appealed to the doctors' and nurses' pay review body. Strange, because the doctors this body covers are hospital doctors. GPs are outside its remit because they are private contractors and not NHS employees. Suddenly and oddly, in this quest for money, GPs became quasi employees. Perhaps it is time they became actual employees and then when prescribing guidelines come from regulatory bodies, they would at least know they were being issued by agencies of their employers and not mere colleagues. Whatever happened to the idea the public still fondly imagines exists—the selfless calling?

The new contract which the most influential trade union in the country, the BMA negotiated, without the primary interests of patients uppermost in their minds, has not made for progress. An article on this subject in The Independent in July 2006 said:

"Do doctors care? Not a lot. Mine didn't think twice about excluding me, even though I have a serious heart condition. Doctors know full well that patients find the changes they've made to the appointments system unworkable. But they weren't devised for our convenience. They were devised to extract as much money as possible out of the new contract. GPs need to ditch the answer-phones, extend availability, employ more staff and make patients feel valued. They're rapidly spending their quota of goodwill among the British public and it's high time we let the Government know. The system isn't working, so fix it, or build a new one."

Benzodiazepine patients have much experience of the caring nature of medicine. In 'The Tranquilliser Trap', an experience far from uncommon was described. A patient told of the medical reaction when the possibility of the pills doing harm was raised:

"Oh he just went mad. He just...he was pointing his finger at me and sort of like holding me and pointing his finger at me and telling me that he knew and I didn't know anything about anything and he just got really, really angry. And I took a book in with me to say that I'd read it here and everything and he said "Put your stupid book away" and everything."

Things said by doctors in connection with benzodiazepines have been assiduously collected by Ray Nimmo of benzo.org.uk. Here are some of them:

"This drug is perfectly safe."

"You have been off Xanax for a month now. Because of its short half life you could not possibly be still experiencing withdrawal symptoms."

"This must be due to some underlying psychological problem. I am going to switch you to Klonopin."

"I am the doctor here."

"You heard about this on the internet???"

"The worst of the withdrawals should be over in about three days. If you're no better in a week, see your GP and he'll give you something. In the meantime get some sleep—you look terrible." (Young UK Casualty doctor)

"You're having a difficult time because you are too sensitive to medication!"

"Take two, they're small."

"So, you say you are feeling better after tapering Xanax...the Xanax wasn't making you feel bad to begin with...you have simply "re-wired" your brain."

"People with anxiety disorders cannot become dependent upon benzodiazepines."

"The withdrawal will be over within two weeks—tops."

"You are feeling agitated; restless and you can't sit still or concentrate? I am changing your diagnosis to manic depression."

"Why do you even bother to read that internet trash and upset yourself?"

"You will never be able to function without Xanax. You cannot handle absolute reality."

"It's impossible to get addicted to something that your body really needs."

On Xanax: "Don't worry about addiction. Because you are on such a low dose for your size and weight, addiction will never be an issue."

"If you take it every day on schedule you won't have to worry about addiction."

"Yes, I might have heard some depression could be possible, so I'm going to write you a prescription..."

"I can't help you if you don't take your medicine."

"Some people just have to take a little all the time." (Psychiatrist)

> "It can't be from withdrawal, it's been two weeks. He must have developed a seizure disorder."

> "You could take it (this small amount) for fifty years and never get addicted."

> "I've never heard anything like it. I've never heard of anyone having so much trouble with benzodiazepines! Most people just have the *jitters* for about two weeks and that's it."

> "These drugs are so good that I would like to see them put in the water. That way everyone can enjoy the benefit of them."

These were collected in the VOT (Victims of Tranquillisers) Newsletter August 1995, First and Last Issue:

> "Your problem is because you were born in the blitz."

> "Your problem is because you were born in a thunderstorm."

> "These pills are OK, it's only the blue ones that are addictive."

> "You'll never see an addict wake up in the night with withdrawal."

> "You will take Valium for the rest of your life or I will not treat you."

> "Go away, I'm striking you off my patients list—I don't want addicts on my register."

These are undoubtedly amusing to read in retrospect, and by the uninvolved, but demonstrate one thing beyond doubt—for a variety of reasons, the depth of expertise among some prescribers on the subject of psychotropic drugs cannot be measured with a micrometer. As Nicholas Regush, Emmy-nominated investigative medical and science journalist wrote in 2002:

> "Medicine as we know it is dying...The disease is caused by conflict of interest, tainted research, greed, pretentious doctors and scientists, lying, cheating...invasion by the morally bankrupt automatons of the drug industry, derelict politicians and...regulators."

And what doctors want for themselves is rather different to what the ordinary mortal is expected to receive:

> "One in three NHS doctors has so little faith in the Health Service they would rather be treated privately according to a new survey. The poll for Hospital Doctor magazine also reveals that 22 per cent of doctors in the NHS had actually taken out private medical insurance to avoid being treated on the Health Service."
> Daily Mail, 7 February 2007

Court of Screwed Medicine

"Between them, the Pharmas and their agents, governments and regulators, and doctors and research workers have constructed a 'health-care' system that now seems, almost routinely, to put health second and them on top."
Charles Medawar, Social Audit, January 2007

"When Claudette and I attended the MHRA's focus discussion group on a Seroxat patient information leaflet, the moderator almost jumped down my throat when I mentioned GSK had been done for fraud earlier that year [Elliot Spitzer case 2004]. She actually tried to shush me, and even stepped forward with the appropriate hand signals..."
Stuart A. Jones, Drug Safety Campaigner, July 2007

"It is almost laughable to see the interests of the members of the MHRA. They will all tell us that they are professional people and that they can be regulators at one moment and servants of the pharmaceutical industry the next. However, it is difficult to believe that they can carry out their jobs independently when we look at the relationship of the committee and its sub-committees with the pharmaceutical industry. In the 2002 annual report, seventeen of the thirty four members of the main committee declare personal interests, which include receiving travel expenses and fees, employment as consultants and the ownership of shares. Fourteen declare non-personal interests such as the receipt of research grants.

All the main pharmaceutical companies are represented, from AstraZeneca to Roche and the trend continues through the sub-committees of the Committee on the Safety of Medicines. The Biological sub-committee has eleven members: ten of them declare personal interests and three declare non-personal interests. These interests run to several pages. I do not want to weary the Chamber, but the Chemistry, Pharmacy and Standards committee has fourteen members, seven declaring personal interests and nine declaring non-personal interests. The Pharmacovigilance committee has eight

members: two have declared personal interests and six have declared non-personal interests."
Paul Flynn MP, Westminster Hall Debate on the Medicines and Healthcare Products Regulatory Agency, 10 Nov 2004

In November 2004 the BBC reported that a reform of the way drugs are regulated was being outlined by health ministers to make the system more independent and transparent. A new code of conduct was drawn up for the MHRA, the Department of Health agency which has responsibility for drug licensing. Two lay representatives would sit on the CSM, as well as patient representatives on every advisory group. The proposals were made after years of criticism over conflicts of interest and secrecy within the MHRA. The members of a new body to replace the CSM—the Commission on Human Medicines (CHM), would no longer be able to hold personal interests in the pharmaceutical industry.

Harry Cayton, the government's so-called Patients Tsar, said:

> "I hope that following these reforms the MHRA will be more active in communicating with the public about its processes and decisions."

Richard Brook, Chief Executive of MIND wondered though:

> "...whether any of this would have come about without the huge amount of public pressure and negative publicity around drug companies' inappropriate behaviour with regards to the aggressive promotion of certain antidepressants."

Health Minister Lord Warner also said it was important that the MHRA was:

> "...open and transparent."

He said the changes meant that:

> "...everyone can be confident in the impartial and independent expert advice given on the safety of medicines."

But is that statement of optimism in any way justified?

NERO—"no evidence of risk is evidence of no risk" and NOROSE—"no research into an adverse reaction is evidence of no adverse reaction", are acronyms which all too accurately describe the intellectual thinking of drug regulators and are an observable measure of the scientific rigour behind their pronouncements on harm. And given the traditional medical view of the value of patient reporting—i.e. it is anecdotal and therefore inferior to scientific reports, it is quite reasonable to have doubts about whether regulators will change that stance following the introduction of patient reporting.

In addition, if for a variety of reasons, patient reports on drugs such as SSRIs and benzodiazepines do not flood in, does that mean the drugs are safe and patients are happy with them? Probably not. The reality is that most patients trust the doctor when he says a medicine is safe and trust the information leaflet when it says a medicine is safe. So if anything untoward happens, those are the sources patients will normally go to for reassurance that the medicine is not at fault. For these reasons alone the regulator would be wise to view the numbers of reports from patients with scepticism—an attitude they should have employed in evaluating the numbers and nature of reactions reported by doctors through the Yellow Card system.

The UK regulators, the CSM/CHM and the MHRA believe in figures rather than patient safety. In 1980 the predecessor of the CSM/CHM, the Committee on the Review of Medicines, in its 'Systematic Review of the Benzodiazepines' concluded that:

> "The number dependent on benzodiazepines in the UK from 1960 to 1977 has been estimated at twenty-eight persons. This is equivalent to a dependence rate of 5–10 cases per million patient months."

It has long been known that the agency estimate was a complete nonsense, so where did the figure come from? The figure came from adding up the total number of Yellow Cards sent in by doctors during that period i.e. 28 and creating a ratio between that number and the number of prescriptions issued.

What effect did that view have on doctors who were prescribing the drugs, which according to the CRM were extremely unaddictive and had very few side-effects? This must certainly have reinforced the same message being disseminated directly to doctors by the benzodiazepine manufacturers. It was the patient who suffered by this totally unscientific message from the Regulator. It extended the scale of harm, and projected it forward in time, and it is likely it added to later denial and the desire to hide the true impact of benzodiazepines on patients.

Benzodiazepines replaced barbiturates and here is another example of the focus of regulators on numbers. By the 1970s in the UK, there were 20,000 emergency hospital admissions due to barbiturate poisoning, which included some 2000 deaths. These were large figures and the drugs were obviously far from safe. Roche embarked on a campaign of persuasion to replace barbiturates with benzodiazepines because the latter were **much safer in overdose**. But deaths through overdose it was later found, was the only way in which the drugs were safer. The comparative death ratios were the key motivating factor, used by Roche, to convince regulators and doctors that benzodiazepines were safe drugs. And once licensed as safe drugs with 'few side-effects', the sales campaign to doctors was so intense and successful, that during the five years from 1978 to 1982, 150 million prescriptions were issued in the UK.

At the end of October 2005, when the CSM became part of the new Commission on Human Medicines, under the new code Commissioners were precluded from holding personal interests in the pharmaceutical industry. That certainly was desirable progress but **how much** progress is debatable.

Sociologists now talk of regulatory capture by the pharmaceutical industry. The revolving door is an important element in that capture. In a November 2004 debate on the UK drugs regulator, Melanie Johnson, the Parliamentary Under-Secretary of State for Health said:

> "I will make a point about the agency's relationship with industry that I believe hon. Members will be keen to hear. The working relationship that the agency needs to have with industry does not inhibit the scientific and regulatory independence of the MHRA...a significant proportion of the MHRA's senior scientific staff are, of course, recruited from, or have a history in, the industry. That is necessary, as they make up the largest single pool of specialist advice for effective drug regulation. They must be drawn from the industry; there is no other source. We need to accept that the pool of people who may have a background in the drugs industry and who understand how it works are likely to be from the industry. The question is where Members believe we would acquire experts who at no point in their past have some sort of background connected with the drugs industry. We will bring UK policy into line with the new EU legislation on these matters which requires that experts should have no financial or other interest in the pharmaceutical industry that could affect their impartiality."

The assertion that only those people with previous pharmaceutical industry experience are capable of policing it, has to be a complete nonsense, and has much more to do with the cosy working relationship between the Department of Health as a whole, the drugs Regulator and the Pharmaceutical Companies. The belief put forward that only those with a drug company working history can understand the evidence presented by manufacturers is facile, particularly since it transpires that the Regulator does not routinely work on raw data but rather on summaries provided by the industry.

John Abraham, Professor of Sociology at the University of Sussex, made these comments in the Guardian in 2005:

> "There is too much of a revolving door syndrome at the MHRA. Not only do CSM members take fees from industry, but many agency officials used to work for drug companies. I would suggest, to a lay person there is a big problem with the concept of independence from industry of a body that is fully funded by industry. The criticism of the old Department of Health medicines department in the 70s was that it didn't have any teeth. Not only does it not now have any teeth, but it is not motivated to bite."

Personal financial interests in the drugs industry are now prohibited, bringing the UK into line with Europe, but that element was never the only factor in the influence of the pharmaceutical industry on regulators. In March 2003, Sarah Bosely, in the Guardian, wrote an article entitled, 'Drugs inquiry thrown into doubt over members' links with manufacturers'. The article examined the subject of a proposed inquiry into the affair of antidepressant SSRIs. As it said:

> "The credibility of a government inquiry intended to settle the controversy surrounding widely prescribed antidepressant drugs was thrown into question yesterday by revelations that most of the members have shareholdings or other links to the manufacturers."

Those with interests in SSRIs but not part of the charmed circle were rightly unhappy with both the membership of the inquiry and with the role of the expert witnesses. Two of the four proposed CSM members were holders of shares in GlaxoSmithKline, the manufacturers of Seroxat. They were Michael Donaghy, a reader in clinical neurology at the University of Oxford, and David Nutt, a professor of psychopharmacology at Bristol University. In some sort of mannered dance, to demonstrate impartiality, the usual convention was to be used and because of their financial stake they would leave the room when Seroxat was discussed. Then, having changed partners as it were, they would re-enter for the debate on SSRIs in general.

The Department of Health and the drugs regulators themselves have always maintained that it is sufficient for members to declare their interests in drug companies before meetings and to leave the room if they have personal interests such as shareholdings. They now maintain that it is perfectly possible and reasonable for us to believe that careers in drug companies and/or research funding from drug companies, exerts no influence on their decisions and views on drug safety. The view put forward whenever criticisms are made is always something along the lines of—'the system for preventing conflicts of interest works well; committee members and members of working groups are professionals of the highest standing in their fields and there is no evidence that members have acted other than with propriety and integrity.'

One expert witness, Dr Baldwin did declare a personal interest in Lundbeck, the makers of Citalopram. But according to the minutes, he did not declare his connections with five other companies, including Seroxat manufacturers GlaxoSmithKline. His department had been funded by SmithKline Beecham, Bristol-Myers Squibb, Eli Lilly, Organon, and Pharmacia for studies by the same five companies and he had been paid by them for speaking at symposia to other doctors about the drugs.

Benzodiazepine activists have come across Professor Nutt many times before. In the past, in his role as chairman of a Home Office drugs advisory committee, he rejected campaigner calls for the reclassification of benzodiazepines as Class A drugs, partly on the grounds that to do so would unnecessarily make life more difficult for illegal users of the drug. He seemed unimpressed by the fact that the calls were being made in an attempt to curb legal prescriptions. Professor Nutt has said he believes that benzodiazepines can be used quite safely by psychiatrists and holds minority views on their health impact. In July 2004 he told the Independent that anti-drug addiction vaccines for children were likely to be among his panel's recommendations when it reported in 2005. He said:

> "People can be vaccinated against drugs at birth as you are against measles."

Nutt and the invited expert on SSRIs, David Baldwin, Senior Lecturer in Psychiatry at Southampton University, both fronted the GSK promotional press launch of Seroxat after it was given a licence by the MHRA to be prescribed for social anxiety disorder, a condition which many doubt even exists as an illness. The chairman of the SSRI inquiry was set to be Angus Mackay, a director of mental health services in Scotland. Mackay was one of the signatories to an influential (and as it turned out, grossly inaccurate) paper produced by the CSM in 1996 which concluded that withdrawal symptoms from SSRIs are:

> "...rare, relatively mild and do not have the features of a physical drug dependency syndrome."

On 28 June 2006 Dr Aubrey Blumsohn, a researcher at Sheffield University, sent an email to Susan Kramer, Liberal Democrat MP for Richmond Park, and Steve Webb, MP Liberal Democrat Shadow Health Secretary. He had vainly attempted to get access to the data from a research project that he was ostensibly leading, and to control the writing of research abstracts that were done supposedly by him. His attempts were opposed by Procter & Gamble, the company that made the drug he was studying and who had paid for the research. Answering points made by the politicians he said:

> "Doctors, researchers, and authors fronting scientific papers about pharmaceuticals are [also] being denied information about the drugs they are prescribing, and manipulated "scientific" material is being written by companies as if it derived from University academics (such as myself). The regulators are seemingly accepting the information fed to them by companies with blind faith—with demonstrably catastrophic results...The whole structure of science in pharmaceutical medicine has failed, and the MHRA is certainly implicated in and has colluded with this failure."

The MHRA replaced or merged with the Medical Devices Agency and the Medicines Control Agency on 1 April 2003. The aim of the new agency, it was said, was to ensure that medicines sold or supplied in the United Kingdom, were of an acceptable standard of safety, quality and efficacy. It also had a responsibility to promote the safe use of medicines and devices. The drugs agency may have acquired a new name but the philosophy did not change. There were concerns from the start about the continuing underlying problems in the organisation and how it works. In the Westminster Hall debate in November 2004, Dr Ian Gibson, head of the Commons Science and Technology Committee described the agency as a:

> "...disaster waiting to happen."

Professor Kent Woods, the Chief Executive of the MHRA had told the Commons Health Committee that:

> "Our prime responsibility is to ensure we protect public health."

But protecting public health, like much health speak today, seems to have two different meanings, depending on whether you talk to those affected or those whose job it is to see that iatrogenic injury is minimised. Reports in the press regarding damage done by benzodiazepines and now SSRIs, have not led to prompt inquiry and measures to reduce the scale of the harm that was being reported. Rather, something of the opposite happens. The agency emphasises that millions have been helped by the drug, that panic among patients must not be stimulated and that ongoing scrutiny of the drugs is taking place. It must be allowed to base its decisions on balanced benefit/risk judgements, and would any patients claiming to have been harmed, plus the media who are channelling their reports of injury, and over-zealous politicians, please recognise that reality. Basically a message of 'trust us.'

In 2004 the Canadian Pharmacists' Association produced a data sheet for Ativan (lorazepam). The sheet warned that lorazepam causes excessive sedation at standard doses, so no one taking it should drive or use heavy machinery. It also specifically warned that Ativan should not be used initially for more than a week, prescriptions should not be automatically renewed, and withdrawal symptoms could appear after as little as a week. The sheet added:

> "Use of benzodiazepines, including lorazepam, may lead to potentially fatal respiratory depression."

What did the Regulator do to fulfil its prime responsibility of protecting public health in the UK? In short it did nothing. Professor Ashton in a letter to Phil Woolas said:

> "The Canadian data sheet includes a warning that benzodiazepines, including lorazepam, may lead to potentially fatal respiratory depression, a statement not present in the current UK data sheet. This variation was approved by the MHRA according to Sir Alasdair's letter, but the UK Ativan data sheet has not been amended—there is no revision of text in the latest data sheet. When will the Canadian warning appear in the UK data sheet? The Canadian data sheet recommends that the initial course of treatment with Ativan should last no longer than one week without reassessment, while the UK data sheet suggests that treatment can vary from a few days to four weeks before re-evaluation. Another difference is that the smallest UK tablet of lorazepam is 1mg, while 0.5mg tablets are available in Canada. These two discrepancies could lead to important and potentially dangerous differences in prescribing practices. Dependence on benzodiazepines, including Ativan, can develop within two weeks and is almost inevitable after 4 weeks of regular use. Furthermore, the likelihood of dependence is increased with higher doses. Thus the "suggested" UK treatment of patients

for up to four weeks, using 1mg lorazepam tablets (each equivalent to 10mg of diazepam (Valium) could well result in a further generation of benzodiazepine-dependent patients, the dangers of which have been fully reported elsewhere, and possibly further benzodiazepine-related deaths. It could also lead to further leakage of benzodiazepines into the illicit drug scene, since much of the illicit benzodiazepine market is derived from doctors' prescriptions. This question should also be pursued with the relevant committees and the Recommendations made consistent. The risks should also be incorporated into Patients' Information Leaflets."

On 3 October 2004, the BBC in the Panorama programme, 'Taken on Trust', looked at the subject of the SSRI antidepressant Seroxat, produced by GlaxoSmithKline. It asked whether the MHRA had acted responsibly in protecting patients. GSK declined to be interviewed on the question of whether they had been aware of the danger Seroxat posed to children but they assured the programme that they themselves had only been aware of the danger since May 2003 after a review of their trials data, and had then acted promptly to inform the Regulator. The significant point was, however, that the subsequent decision of the Regulator to prohibit use of Seroxat with children was based on three depression trials, the last of which had ended in 2001. Professor Breckenridge, the MHRA head was asked if GSK had acted promptly in his opinion. He said:

> "This is a matter which we are investigating at the present time. There is an investigation going on, being conducted by the inspection and enforcement sector of the agency and with lawyers to decide whether or not they did."

Did he think two years was an acceptable delay because during that time children were being prescribed a drug now known to be harmful? The MHRA, he said, had acted with great rapidity—within two weeks of receiving the information. But to the question of why the MHRA apparently had not been able to acquire the information earlier, he had no real answer, other than to repeat that it was being investigated. There might possibly be criminal charges, but to date none have been brought. When the MHRA announced the Seroxat children's ban in 2003, it said the ban was based on new information but Richard Brook of MIND said this was misleading:

> "I felt that the MHRA seemed to suggest that it was new information to them and to Glaxo and that I didn't think was fair, and I had several discussions after the press conference

on the very day with the head of post-licensing expressing my concern. We had a meeting subsequently and in the end we were told that it would be looked at criminally and the only thing that we did to raise the issues would be in breach of the procedures and the law that surrounded these sorts of things. In other words we were warned off about making a fuss about it."

The MHRA Expert Working Group (May 2003–March 2004), on which Brook sat as an invited member, asked GlaxoSmithKline to re-analyse its original clinical trial results. When they did, they found evidence to suggest that eighteen to twenty-nine year olds could be at an increased risk of suicidal behaviour. This information had taken thirteen years to discover. Was the information presented but not analysed? That was a question, the MHRA chairman assured us, which was also under investigation. As interviewer Shelley Jofre said:

> "Panorama can reveal that this current review is the first time the raw data from the original clinical trials has been properly analysed."

She went on to say:

> "The information about young adults was in the original trial data given to the Regulator in the late 80s. So how could it have missed such an important signal? The answer may lie in the licensing process. The MHRA takes an awful lot on trust when it makes its decisions about a medicine's safety. Each clinical trial produces a huge amount of information and this raw data is summarised by the drug companies. The Regulator then relies on these summaries. It rarely studies the raw data itself. With the SSRIs however, there have been five safety reviews since 1991. Each one of these was an opportunity to spot what was missed originally."

Charles Medawar and Dr Andrew Herxheimer have pointed out that none of these reviews examined all the raw data from GSK either. Asked how rigorous the previous reviews of the SSRI antidepressants were, Richard Brook said:

> "...sitting here in 2004, they are not really worth the paper they're written on. The reasons for that are quite complex but basically it seems that they were not robust, they were not

> rigorous and they didn't look at original data, and so they seemed to be as much use as paper in a waste bin."

And the Patient Information Leaflet approved by the Regulator, carried no warning addressed to young adults. The only clue was on the MHRA website from April 2004. All that was said was that doctors should carefully monitor young adults after prescribing Seroxat. Professor Breckenridge gave an assurance that the Patient Leaflet would be altered in due course, following a review, but in the meantime, the information was available on the MHRA website. It did not apparently disturb him that relatively few people, particularly depressed people, are likely to scour the site for information. Richard Brook said:

> "The Regulator may well have created a situation where people have died. It makes me very sad for the families and the people that I've got to know during this time dealing with Seroxat..."

Those who are knowledgeable about the history of benzodiazepines and their regulation were not surprised by any of this. Quoting from Hansard, 5 March 1980, Charles Medawar said this in his book 'Power and Dependence':

> "Mr Carter-Jones asked the Secretary of State for Social Services what study his department had made of possible addictions to Valium.
> Dr Vaughan: The Committee on the Review of Medicines (CRM), with an expert sub-committee including eminent psychiatrists, has made a comprehensive study of all aspects of the clinical use of benzodiazepines, including diazepam, the active ingredient of Valium. On the basis of present knowledge the CRM has concluded that addiction potential was generally low..."

As the Seroxat programme pointed out, Richard Brook had exposed major failings in the UK system of medicines regulation. He had found that for years the MHRA missed crucial safety evidence on Seroxat, a failure which should raise concerns about other medicines. As Brook commented:

> "I have little confidence that the drugs they're licensing day by day are being licensed in a way I would feel appropriate and what's even more concerning I have very little confidence in drugs that have been regulated in the past."

When GSK applied for a licence for child use, the Regulator had discovered for the first time that the company's own clinical trial data revealed that the drug did not work in depressed children. More than that, it made them up to three times more likely to self harm and attempt suicide than depressed children who were given placebos. Richard Brook said:

> "It was really a shock to them. In discussions directly with me, officials were saying we have defended this drug for a decade. There has never been a sign as far as we're concerned about an issue here, and suddenly we're faced with this. And as that story unfolded it becomes clearer and clearer that the sort of way the information is put into the MHRA's possession, all of that is somewhat suspect to say the least."

Dr David Healy explained:

> "The data that went in from the clinical trials on these drugs done fifteen to twenty years ago makes it absolutely clear when you add the whole thing up that actually the rates at which people become suicidal on these drugs—and this isn't just children or young adults, this is any age group at all, is two and a half times greater on the drug than it is in people taking placebo."

How much value should be placed on the statement from Professor Breckenridge that the primary role of the MHRA is to protect the public's health, and that it has a responsibility to ensure that only drugs which are effective and safe come to the market and remain on the market? Dr Healy said:

> "Back when I approached the Regulator first at the end of 1999 I thought this is an issue that could have been sorted out with him in some months. I guess pretty well every year for the last five years I've thought it'll get sorted this year. But it's still not sorted."

After nearly half a century, the damage benzodiazepine addiction does to patients who have trusted medicine is still 'not sorted.'

The fact that those steeped in the culture of drugs and their benefit rather than their risk, never really move their thinking into a new perspective, was very clearly illustrated by Professor Breckenridge's determination to salvage a picture of large benefit and little harm for the major area of Seroxat use—those over the age of thirty. Dr Healy **might**

have been right about the harm posed to children but he was **definitely not right** in regard to adults over thirty. Breckenridge used as justification for his expert opinion a recent analysis of three hundred clinical trials—all funded by GlaxoSmithKline which not surprisingly proved the drug safe for use in adults over thirty. No alarm bells that the studies had all been funded by the manufacturer? Apparently there were not.

> "There is very good clinical trial evidence that these drugs do not cause suicide, they do not cause suicidal thoughts in adults. There is a very large database."

Professor Peter Tyrer, Head of Psychological Medicine, Imperial College, London, disagrees:

> "I think the evidence that these tablets can cause suicidal feelings is now absolutely clear. I don't think really we can dispute it..."

Interestingly, Peter Tyrer has been proved right in the past. In a Lancet report in 1981, around the same time as the Regulator was declaring that benzodiazepine addiction was very rare indeed, he showed that between a quarter and a half of the patients studied, who had taken lorazepam or diazepam for four months or more, had withdrawal symptoms and were judged to have been 'pharmacologically dependent' on the drugs they took. At that time, massive numbers of prescriptions were being issued and large numbers of people had been taking the drugs longer than four months—a sizeable proportion, very much longer.

Regulators seem not to understand safety or speed as those concepts are understood by the public, rather they lapse into the language of the controlling and not the protector. Breckenridge's view on who owns the meaning of drug safety and makes the decisions is typical. It may be the public health which is affected but it is the Regulator who decides how much it is affected and whether to act. This has an air of fascism about it:

> "It is a matter of regulatory and practical judgement as to when information should be transmitted. When it is in the public's interest that information should be transmitted rapidly, we will do it."

This statement reflects the arrogance of the regulatory establishment and not their expertise. The data on Seroxat which the Regulator had held for thirteen years demonstrated categorically that Seroxat had little benefit above a 20mg dosage. And the side-effects, particularly around withdrawal, increased quite dramatically post 20mg but Breckenridge was in no hurry to let the public know that.

Richard Brook, not surprisingly, felt the public **should** know and was eventually forced into a position where he said that if the MHRA would not tell the public, then he would do so. The response of the Court of Screwed Medicine, the purported protector of patient health, was to threaten him with legal action if he made any kind of unauthorised disclosure. This was a position it could not maintain and the Regulator eventually did write to doctors explaining the findings of the working group. But in the surreal world of regulation, reputation is all and so the findings were presented to the prescribers as a reminder. The fact that the information was completely new to doctors and not a reminder at all, disturbed the MHRA not one jot. They said that after reviewing the drug extensively, they felt a reminder was in order. This was very far from honest. Naturally, there was no admission that the information about dosage had been around for thirteen years and they had not, as experts on drug safety, noticed it.

Seroxat became the most profitable drug that GlaxoSmithKline has ever made and the controversy about its effects did not stop that. It became, just as benzodiazepines did, a triumph of marketing over science. As Professor Tyrer has commented:

> "For a time, even only in a matter of a few years, almost [all] critical scepticism [and] objectivity was suspended in favour of the all out rush to develop these new drugs and develop new markets."

Substitute Librium, Valium, Mogadon and the whole host of other benzodiazepines—the 'original and best' and the me-too copies, for Seroxat, and you have a parallel story being played over once again. More than that, it is a story being repeated while the original story has still not reached the final chapter.

Professor Tyrer knew something about benzodiazepines and he knows something about Seroxat. GSK employed Peter Tyrer as a world expert on drug dependence, to conduct their clinical trial into the drug's effects on depressed patients in the late 1980s. During those trials he discovered, as he had with lorazepam and diazepam ten years earlier, that patients could become dependent. After six weeks on Seroxat some of his patients were feeling better, but some of them could not stop the drug:

> "After the trial ended they said: "Can we continue on these tablets because we feel we've got to have them because they seem to be so effective", but more concerning...was...more concerning to us was the fact that they were saying: "I cannot tolerate the symptoms when I stop it"."

Some of the withdrawal effects were not those found in patient leaflets, or warned about by the MHRA. Trial volunteers had, as Professor Tyrer described, feelings of dysphoria, the feeling of being depressed and in some cases were entertaining suicidal thoughts. These results were passed to GSK but Tyrer found that the manufacturer did not seem very interested. Tyrer does not believe that GSK ever investigated the problem. Perhaps they preferred instead to accentuate the positive.

Had the regulators been aware of the problem? If they were aware, like GSK, they preferred to stress the plus aspects—this in spite of the fact that after licensing, the drug attracted more Yellow Card reports on withdrawal problems than any other prescription drug. Turning the world on its head, Breckenridge preferred to state that patients held all the responsibility:

> "They were warned from the time the drug was licensed that there was a risk of withdrawal. This has been mentioned in every review, every publication coming from the Committee on Safety of Medicines, the problem of withdrawal, that has been publicised in patient information leaflets that there is a problem with withdrawal."

Like much else that the Regulator says, it was not true. Patients were not aware and neither were their doctors. Until 2003 the Patient Leaflet was saying that withdrawal symptoms were "not common" and "you cannot become addicted to Seroxat". The wording was approved by the Regulator.

Where does informed consent enter a situation when the Regulator, the Patient Leaflets it approves, and prescribing doctors, tell those who take the drug that the risk of withdrawal symptoms is slight? As Peter Tyrer said, the patient would have understood from the information presented to them, that their risk of dependency was low and that when they stopped taking the drug they would have no problem with that process. But as he also pointed out, the evidence did not support that message. Sarah Venn of the Seroxat Users Group told the BBC:

> "I am absolutely fuming that this drug was allowed to be put on the market with completely misleading information that people like me were taking it, believing what we were told, doctors believing what they were being told. There is no reason why I should be sitting here today in the state that I am because the regulators knew about this problem. GlaxoSmithKline knew about this problem, but they did nothing and they have changed the course of my life and thousands of other lives."

Richard Brook says it is clear from the information that he saw, that the original Seroxat trial data demonstrated there were quite severe withdrawal issues, that there was no mistaking the meaning. It was very clear that withdrawal affected people significantly, particularly at higher dosages and at long periods of using the drug. The information showing these realities had been held by the MHRA for over a decade and had been known to the manufacturer even longer than that.

More than a decade after this information was acquired by the MHRA, in June 2003 the Patient Leaflet changed radically. The claim about a small likelihood of dependence disappeared to be replaced by something quite different. Suddenly patients were being told that one in four people could now experience withdrawal problems and some of these could be more severe than the symptoms which took them to the doctor in the first place. In the view of the Regulator however, twelve years to make patients aware of the new views on safety was not too long a period of time. In the opinion of Professor Breckenridge:

> "It takes time for clinical trial evidence to become available."

Obviously, what the everyman understands by protection is not what the Regulator understands. As Charles Medawar told 'Taken on Trust':

> "The Regulator should be covered in shame to admit that they had failed to spot an adverse effect which people had been sounding off about on the internet in their thousands and thousands, and suddenly to admit that this side effect is real after all and that it affects a quarter of all users. The Regulator should be deeply ashamed."

Since the drug was licensed, patients and their families and some doctors had tried to tell the Regulator about dependence, about self harm, about the risk to children and about the risk of suicide. Had the Regulator listened? It seems they did not, since even after the overwhelming evidence outlined in the Panorama programmes on Seroxat, Breckenridge was still manfully fighting his corner and declaring that no regulatory agency in the world had done more to keep SSRI drugs under scrutiny. He seemed to feel no sense of irony in maintaining that that was what the MHRA had done and would continue to do—in the 'interests of public health.'

The media tends to look at the problems surrounding drugs, one drug at a time, but we should be concerned about the performance of the Regulator on all drugs. Benzodiazepine-injured patients and campaigners hold that to be a self-evident truth. For decades they have been fighting a battle to get the Department of Health and its agencies to do something effective about the scale of damage, but so far it has not happened. The Regulator has no power or responsibility to enforce guidelines patients are told, and the Department of Health wilfully maintains, in the face of incontrovertible evidence to the contrary, that it is patients who abuse the drugs rather than the drugs which abuse the patient. As Richard Brook said:

> "I think this is actually an issue that probably goes beyond Seroxat and I find it hard not to believe there aren't other drugs that might be in the same category as Seroxat, that have lacked that robust clear analysis that has allowed us to make a decision about how they should be used—what information people need before they use them. So I actually think this is a major issue for us in the UK."

Dr Mike Shooter, former President of the Royal College of Psychiatrists, agrees with him:

> "I think once again we're seeing the SSRIs being the focus for something much wider in psychiatry and we're seeing psychiatry being the focus for something much, much wider in medicine as a whole. I think, you know, a few years down the line we're going to be talking about this with many more sorts of medication than psychotropic medication."

This letter from the MHRA to the author in March 2004 illustrates the degree of seriousness the Regulator attaches to patient reporting:

> Your letter has been passed to the MHRA (Medicines and Healthcare products Regulatory Agency) for reply, as the agency responsible for the safety, quality and efficacy of licensed medicines.
>
> In your letter you have raised concerns which have been addressed in previous correspondence and new concerns which I will address in this reply.
>
> You have raised the possibility that patients may be educated in prescription drug safety to improve appropriate prescribing. Patients currently receive information in Patient Information Leaflets (PILS) and consideration is being given as to how to improve communication, especially the concept of risk/benefit.
>
> The MHRA cannot comment on the adequacy of service provision for patients with benzodiazepine addiction since

> this remit is the concern of the wider department, however, we will share your concerns with our colleagues in the wider department
> Pharmacovigilance Risk Assessment Unit

This was the letter I had sent to the Health Minister, dated 2nd December 2003:

> Dear Rosie Winterton
> At your recent meeting with Benzact, Beat the Benzos and Professor Ashton, you mentioned that new NICE advice to doctors would be available in the New Year. Welcome as this is, you will be aware, as Professor Appleby (Mental health Director at the Department of Health) has given an opinion, that Guidelines are not enough. The history of the benzodiazepines since 1988 has clearly demonstrated that for reasons not related to improvement of patient health, doctors have continued to prescribe well beyond what is clinically sound.
> Professor C.H. Ashton through her work on benzodiazepines has estimated that there are probably at least a million people addicted in the UK and her Manual indicates the kind of symptoms likely to be experienced in withdrawal. Professor Malcolm Lader has said that in some unknown way, drugs such as diazepam seem to become ingrained and with a significant proportion of former patients having their health following withdrawal severely damaged for the long-term.
> This reality is not reflected in information supplied to doctors by pharmaceutical companies through data sheets. Nor is it reflected in information supplied to doctors centrally by government and their agencies. There are references to withdrawal from tranquillisers taking six weeks. This is a gross under-estimate and probably refers to blood analysis rather than to the observable symptoms. In addition the 200 or so possible side-effects acknowledged recently by the President of the Royal College of Psychiatrists in the BMJ seem to be something of a well kept secret from many GPs.
> The Department of Work and Pensions follows the information provided by the DoH and it is therefore not surprising that people unable to work because of drug effects have to fight for individual recognition. Brain damage, neurological symptoms and blood disorders are all too likely in the long-term addicted but since research into these factors known only to ex-patients

is not funded, it is quite impossible to gain recognition through benefits.

Redress is a very emotive subject with former patients who have been harmed by benzodiazepines. In law, there is basically nothing the damaged can do to gain any kind of compensation. The Legal Aid system is not available as was pointed out recently to the BBC by a Manchester law firm. When the No-Win-No Fee system was introduced in 1991 after Legal Aid was reduced, it was intended it was said, to counter-balance a possible denial of access to justice. It has not done this with regard to those harmed by drugs—such people are cut off completely from the legal system. The only course open is to complain to your doctor—small recompense for lost years and the possibility of permanent health damage.

Colin Downes-Grainger, Benzodiazepine Campaigner

The matter of drug safety is played out like a game at the Court of Screwed Medicine. Did the Pharmacovigilance Unit share the concerns with the wider department? Who knows? But one thing is very certain, the 'wider department' has been well aware of the concerns for a long time and the official response has not changed for years. You may start out believing that the Regulator and the Department of Health will react positively to reasoned argument and a demonstration of the real impact of licensed drugs but in the face of continuing avoidance tactics, non-logic, untruth and deliberate misunderstanding, that optimism quickly dissipates.

The MHRA has a reputation for not giving out information and it remains to be seen whether the new commitment to 'transparency' enables those outside the system to truly examine how well that system is working. It will take more than a redesigned website and the appointment of a communications director to deal with the traditional culture of secrecy. The Department of Health seems determined to preserve as much of the past as possible in spite of the fact that the past system has killed and injured enormous numbers of people.

"The FDA is in a shambles, and there is considerable evidence that Britain's Medicines and Healthcare Regulatory Agency is not in any better shape..."

David Healy, Letter to British Medical Journal, 29 July 2006

"Drug regulators too, seem unequal to their task. Critics focus on their close relationship with industry; their lack of transparency; their lack of systematic post marketing surveillance; and an emphasis on efficacy over patient safety, which favours industry..."

Fiona Godlee, Editor, BMJ, 8 July 2006

When the Government announced direct reporting by consumers, Charles Medawar was not the only sceptic. MIND stated what has become obvious when it said:

> "Consumer representation and the championing of consumer rights is not built into the MHRA's structures and processes."

There is a need for a legal requirement to protect genuinely sensitive market information, but there is more than a suspicion that the MHRA and the DoH use this requirement to avoid disclosure in areas which have nothing at all to do with commercial confidentiality. In an open society and particularly in medicine which is after all concerned with the improvement and protection of health, sharing information is of prime importance.

A working drug regulatory system should put consumer safety before commercial pressure and cost. In such a system the MHRA would insist on access to all trial results. They would insist that this information, without restrictions, should be available to researchers and reviewers and, once a drug is licensed, that the information was made available to all. If this required clarification of the law or its amendment, a drug agency truly concerned with the protection of citizens would pressure government to provide the changes needed.

It is not enough that regulators have no personal interest in the industry that they are reviewing and regulating. There should be a majority of people regulating drugs who are not linked to drug companies through research or other career dependencies. If David Healy, when allowed access to SSRI data, can immediately understand its importance and its variance from the drug company line of universal benefit, how is it possible to view the statement of health minister Melanie Johnson that there is no other source of regulatory personnel than the pharmaceutical industry—other than with incredulity and suspicion? Does the MHRA have too many hats and not enough heads? Who does it really serve? The experience of campaigners, who know what they are talking about, suggests that its priorities are more aligned with its financiers than protecting those on the receiving end of the medicines those financiers provide.

In a world where information is restricted, it is hard to make criticisms stick, and that, you might believe, is a handy weapon to have in the face of criticism. Assurances and statements of benefit are the regulator's stock in trade. But unless you have made a detailed study of the contrasts between the statements and the impact of drugs in the real world, then you are in no position to judge. Paul Flynn, an MP who is more aware than most politicians of the failures in the regulatory system, the influence of the pharmaceutical industry and the consequences of those things, said in the parliamentary debate on the MHRA:

> "Recent events have proven that [the MHRA] is not a watchdog—it is a pussycat that purrs in front of the pharmaceutical industry and does what it is told. It has an incestuous relationship with the Big Pharmas and has a close association with the Association of the British Pharmaceutical Industry. It has a disgraceful recent record...I do not think that the body can be reformed. We have to set up another. We cannot have the public exposed to the greed of the pharmaceutical industry any longer without protection."

He pointed to something which benzodiazepine campaigners know is certainly true when he said:

> "It was not the official watchdog that caused something to be done [on Seroxat]; it was publicity by energetic, intelligent, resourceful journalists—people we often criticise. The real watchdogs are those journalists and organisations such as MIND."

Flynn has become aware, as have many of those who gave evidence to the Parliamentary Health Committee Inquiry into pharmaceutical company influence—that the MHRA has become part of the pharmaceutical industry. It shares its philosophy and its aims.

The pharmaceutical industry has a self-serving record of bending science, of disease-mongering, of hiding negatives and then seeking to influence key figures, in its pursuit of profit. In the US which has a legal system which has been partly able to take on the industry (often very successfully) and a more open approach to disclosure, there are long lists of drug company misdeeds. Questions of the possibility of deceit never seem to enter the consciousness of the UK regulator when it defends its record. As Paul Flynn went on to say:

> "The problems that we now have with selective serotonin reuptake inhibitors reveal how the system has not worked in the interests of patients and how the agency has been colonised by the drugs companies, whose commercial interests have been protected as a result."

It takes about eight weeks to license a drug but it habitually takes a whole lot longer than that for the MHRA to warn consumers about problems discovered and much longer to discover them. Seroxat is a case in point but there are numerous others. One of those concerns was Risperidone, an anti-psychotic drug. It was being used unlicensed in the UK to treat older people with dementia. The Regulator received information in 2002 that the risk of strokes was three times higher among older people prescribed this medication, but it took until 9 March 2004 to warn that the drug should not be used. Patients in Canada had been warned of the risk of strokes two years earlier.

Not only does the MHRA fail to warn but the Regulator believes speedy approval of trials is commensurate with drug safety. In 2005 it declared that it was their target to approve drug trials projects in fourteen days.

In September 2006, the Sunday Times reported on the tragedy of the trial of TGN1412 in six volunteers—one of a new generation of treatments targeting the immune system. The protocol of the trial was approved by the MHRA. The drug was administered on average fifteen times more quickly to the volunteers than it had been to monkeys in earlier animal studies. The speed at which the monkeys received TGN1412 was set out in the trial application to the MHRA by research company Parexel International, acting on behalf of TeGenero, a small German drug developer. The paperwork did not explicitly detail how quickly the volunteers would be given the drug, although it should have been possible to make a calculation from the information provided. The error, later described as crude, led to disastrous consequences.

Apparently, the MHRA had failed to notice that the paperwork from Parexel did not include data on test-tube experiments designed to show the drug's effect on human cells. This was only discovered when the Sunday Times and the Channel 4 Dispatches programme successfully applied under the Freedom of Information Act for the reinstatement of paragraphs cut from documents released by the MHRA.

Experts believe MHRA assessors could have spotted the danger signs if they had taken more time to scrutinise the project. The MHRA of course denied it had missed the warning signs. Understandably, critics are worried that, if the MHRA gave the go-ahead here, in the absence of important information, it could do it again in the future, leading to other avoidable tragedies.

It seems there is very little difference between the approach of the MHRA to evaluation of data provided for licensing applications and its approach to the evaluation of trials applications. And the cutting out of paragraphs which showed clearly the agency's failings in the Parexel trial, illustrated yet again its commitment to self-serving secrecy.

Following the decision of NICE not to approve the Alzheimer's drug Aricept, Dr Paul Hooper, managing director of Eisai Limited, made a comment on the relative influence of patients and Pharma when he said that taking the matter for court review was a last ditch resort. Many drug victims wish they had that ability and opportunity. On 8 January 2007 the judicial review was lodged at the High Court with Pfizer/Eisai as the lead claimant. Whether the NICE decision is flawed is not central to this argument. What is central is the fact that drug companies who do not like the decisions of regulators have the capacity and the resources, to use the law to challenge those decisions. Individual patients do not have the finance to do the same. The ability to look at and challenge the workings behind regulator or watchdog decisions should be far easier than it is for all involved in health, whether as researchers, commentators or patients, but at the present time, it is not open to many to do it, certainly not in the courts or by requesting information and having the request answered. That is the problem.

Interestingly, this is a case of drug companies challenging the decision of a watchdog and insisting that the whole process should be open, but in the case of Seroxat we had an example of a drug company itself apparently being rather less than open. BBC Panorama had interviewed Dr Tim Kendall, Co-Director, Mental Health Guidelines for the National Institute of Clinical Excellence. In 2003, using the published trial data, he and his team were about to recommend that Seroxat and the other SSRIs could be prescribed to children for depression. To assist in the decision they asked the MHRA for the unpublished trial results. When they examined those they found that rather than being an effective treatment, the drug could induce suicide. If NICE had based its decision on the published data, it would have recommended approval and as Dr Kendall said:

> "...there would have been children who might well have killed themselves further down the line as a result of our recommendation. If we can't be sure if there are trials that are being withheld or not published for...you know...sometimes years on end, this absolutely shakes the whole foundation of scientific medicine."

As Mike Shooter observed with an air of shock:

> "I personally felt cheated. Suddenly, the balance between risk and benefit was quite clearly tilted in a different way."

At the House of Commons Health Committee Inquiry on 25 November 2004, Phil Woolas MP was asked to what extent he believed that the drug manufacturers were responsible for the current levels of benzodiazepine use and dependence. He replied:

> "That goes to the nub of the problem. I have referred the Committee to two submissions of written evidence to this

> inquiry...Indeed, as you will know, Mr Chairman, I wrote to you on 13 October of this year suggesting that a number of documents that we have become aware of in our research for legal action in this country and in other countries would show, in my view beyond doubt, that [the]...withholding of the information was intentional [by Wyeth and Roche]."

It seems when it concerns pharmaceutical company interests, conflicting and divergent views on disclosure appear to be perfectly reconcilable with each other. It is very difficult indeed to turn away from a conviction that it is in the relationship between the MHRA and the pharmaceutical industry that the source of the laissez-faire attitude to patient safety can be found. The MHRA listens closely to the concerns of major pharmaceutical companies but it absolutely fails to listen closely to people experiencing side-effects from drugs that should be making them better, not worse. Drug companies have easy access to regulators, as they have to the Department of Health and politicians. Health campaigners on the other hand have virtually no access to decision makers. Concerns are often ignored and when replies are forthcoming, they demonstrate no understanding of what is being said. It is possible to believe that the lack of understanding is deliberate, and centres on the protection of existing systems and individuals.

An enormous rise in prescription drug use in recent years has meant that the pharmaceutical industry has become the third most profitable in the UK, behind tourism and finance—something which the government never ceases to laud in any debate on patient safety.

Beyond the benefit to pharmaceutical shareholders, is the usually uncollated and hidden cost to patients through adverse drug reactions. The former House of Commons Health Committee Chairman, David Hinchliffe, told the BBC in April 2005:

> "The pharmaceutical industry is extremely powerful and influences healthcare at every level. Like any industry, drug companies need effective discipline and regulation, and these have been lacking...The industry, regulator, doctors and other prescribers must take their share of the blame."

It is incredibly hard to pin blame or responsibility on anyone in the UK healthcare system. The energies placed into the avoidance of blame are a major reason why change is so difficult to secure. On the one hand doctors, through Dr Maureen Baker, of the Royal College of GPs, were saying in response to the Health Committee, that GPs act in good faith, have the best interests of patients at heart and had to rely on regulators. But, significantly, on the other hand it was discovered in market research sponsored by the MHRA itself, that four out of ten doctors apparently have no idea who the regulator is, so what value should we place on that statement? And if the regulator is inefficient, or worse, and constantly displays a lack of concern for what the patient understands by patient safety, should doctors be relying on them?

The UK government, through Health Minister Lord Warner has denied that the industry and government are too close. He prefers to stress that the government has an effective and proper working relationship with the pharmaceutical industry. Of course that statement begs the question of what the government means by the word effective. The MHRA has said something similar:

> "The interests of public health are coherent with the promotion of the industry."
> "We do not consider the fee relationship [with drug companies] to be a problem."
> The Guardian, 5 October 2005

And so has the Association of the British Pharmaceutical Industry:

> "The ABPI believes there is a remarkable concordance between the MHRA and our priorities."
> The Guardian, 5 October 2005

In November 2004, Minister Lord Warner, in bowing to pressure and accusations of partiality in the regulatory agencies, described the new government willingness to demonstrate the impartiality of the MHRA and CSM/CHM. He described how in the future, those who sat on the regulatory body would have three months to sell their shares and end consultancy agreements with drug companies. Those who accepted drug company sponsorship, free flights, hotels and restaurant meals from drug companies to attend educational conferences would be barred from committees for six months. But at the same time he reaffirmed the Faith in saying:

> "I don't believe there is a conspiracy between the people who have worked in drug regulation and the industry, **but there is clearly a perception in some quarters that there is a problem. We have to tackle that perception."**

The institutional disbelief was still there.

A Case of Yellow Jaundice

"Reams of discussion and internet traffic have been devoted to the behaviour and attitude of the MHRA, the UK government drug regulatory agency. Many have accused it of colluding with or ignoring industrial scientific fraud, and of severe conflicts of interest. It has been accused of failing to properly examine raw data in drug licensing applications, and of acting against the public interest. Many believe that the actions and omissions of the agency have led to deaths and illness—resulting from undisclosed, delayed or undiscovered information about pharmaceuticals in the UK.
Despite widespread parliamentary, professional and public concern and anger about the MHRA, no meaningful steps have yet been taken by the government to safeguard pharmaceutical science, the public interest or public health..."
Dr Aubrey Blumsohn, June 2006

"And what would I do if a loved one suffered a serious drug reaction? It's virtually impossible to sue a pharmaceutical company in Britain, partly because of the difficulty of getting any funding for such actions. There's no point appealing to the government drugs watchdog—the MHRA. It is a small outfit entirely funded by the drug industry. It has never taken any action against the academics that make fraudulent claims in ghost-written articles, nor doctors working for the companies who repeat such claims, even when they have been shown to be untrue. So the only other body to turn to is the General Medical Council, whose job it is to investigate the conduct of doctors—but it has shown no inclination to act."
Professor David Healy, 6 February 2007

The Yellow Card system is the equivalent to the FDA's MedWatch adverse drug effect reporting system in the US. Both systems have been consistently shown to fail to demonstrate the actual scope and severity of adverse drug reactions after licensing approval and marketing, or to do anything about it in a way that protects patients in a timely fashion. The UK scheme was set up in 1964 after the Thalidomide affair.

Between the years 1963 and 1976, with the ever-increasing millions of benzodiazepine prescriptions being issued each year, doctors sent in 8 Yellow Cards about dependence on benzodiazepines. In recent years the number and proportion of Yellow Cards filed by GPs has decreased from its already unrealistic level. The numbers have been maintained at roughly 20,000 per year only because reporting was extended in later years to coroners, nurses, hospital pharmacists and community pharmacists.

Under-reporting is a feature of our health care system. Indeed, the Minister of State at the Department of Health, Rosie Winterton admitted in a parliamentary answer in April 2004:

> "The number of reports received via the Yellow Card Scheme does not directly equate to the number of people who suffer adverse reactions to drugs for a number of reasons including an unknown level of under-reporting."
> Official Report, 19 April 2004; Vol. 420 c.222W

So how accurate are the estimates of the incidence of adverse reaction reporting and the nature of the reactions? In 'Medicines out of control? Antidepressants and the Conspiracy of Goodwill', 2004, Charles Medawar and Professor Anita Hardon said this:

> "The available evidence suggested that the mythical average doctor reported something closer to around one per cent of the adverse drug reactions (ADRs) there actually were. General Practitioners sent in just under half of all Yellow Cards (9,232 reports from GPs in 2001)—equivalent to about one-third of a Yellow Card per doctor per year."

In the light of this picture, it seems eminently sensible to take much more account of what it is that the **patient** says on the subject of his or her experiences after taking a prescribed drug. This view was expressed clearly at the Health Committee Inquiry in 2004/5:

> "I think ultimately it is difficult to get away from the idea that, difficult though it may be, the best person to tell you about an adverse reaction is the person who is suffering it. That raises a lot of problems for regulators because they say it is very difficult; patients will not be able to understand what a serious effect is, what a minor effect is; it is going to cause a lot of data; there will be a lot of noise in the system; but ultimately, if you want a pure account of what happened and you want to be able to tie that to the taking of a particular medication, the best person to tell you that is the patient. If you rely on a third

party to tell you that, diligent though he or she may be, you start to erode some of the experience. In fact, you may not get the experience if you rely totally on the Yellow Card system."
Dr Ike Iheanacho, Editor, Drug and Therapeutics Bulletin, Evidence to Parliamentary Health Committee, January 2005

"Consumers ought to be filling this up: the work that has been done by Andrew Herxheimer and Charles Medawar on this shows that you get much more information from consumers filling these up. What you might also get if you had that kind of situation, you may also get physicians being more prepared to fill the cards up also and in a more detailed way than they are now."
Professor David Healy, Evidence to Parliamentary Health Committee, January 2005

"Can I also just say that a large number of patients do not manage to succeed in getting their adverse effects reported. That is a consistently big issue for MIND. We have evidence over several years of people trying to report going to their GP, asking for adverse effects to be reported and the GP saying, "I do not think that is actually what has happened and so I am not doing it." I know patient reporting is now starting, but it still, I think, raises a real issue...The other issue that really worries me is the fact that the adverse reporting is seen as very minor in relation to clinical trials, and time after time I have been told that adverse reporting only can give a signal and it is clinical trials that are definitive. I think that is wrong. Those two must be married up."
Richard Brook, Chief Executive of MIND, Evidence to the Parliamentary Health Committee, January 2005

"The other point is that in the Sixties when most of these drugs began to come on stream, the expectation was that physicians would play a role rather like the role they play vis-à-vis tobacco and alcohol, that they would say, "Look, you do not want to believe all the hype that you hear about these things, there may be good uses for them, but they are not always that good." At this point in time one of the biggest problems that we have in the system is the silence of physicians..."
Professor David Healy, Evidence to the Parliamentary Health Committee, January 2005

Doctors and other health professionals are voluntarily supposed to notify watchdogs if a patient reports an "adverse effect". The Yellow Card reporting scheme has been described as the "cornerstone" of the drug regulator's attempts to spot early warning signs that a drug might have previously unknown hazardous side-effects.

You might wonder why it is voluntary. It is possible that when the scheme was devised by Dr Bill Inman, he imagined, after Thalidomide, that doctors would be keen to report adverse reactions and would be keen to make the system for collection of the data work, to prevent any chance of a recurrence. The reality is that it does not happen. The number of reports received each year by the MHRA has remained fairly constant, at around 20,000 since the mid 1980s. Only an estimated 10% of adverse drug reactions are currently reported through the Yellow Card Scheme to the MHRA. It should be said though, that even the often quoted 10% figure is almost meaningless, because the figure varies so much for different reactions and in any case this tentative estimate applied only to 'serious' reactions, with an estimate of only 2–4% for less serious ones. The often quoted reasons for doctors not filling in the adverse reaction reports are these:

- Too busy, put it off, can't find the form and so on.
- Belief in the safety of prescription drugs—echoed in the 2006 Ipsos MORI poll commissioned by the MHRA.
- Guilt about their prescription having done harm.
- Fear of legal come-back, which given the legal system in the UK, is not all that likely.
- Not wishing to be alarmist or appear naive.
- Ignorance of the procedure for reporting—again echoed in the 2006 Ipsos MORI poll.

A good discussion of the low reporting syndrome—including a reference to Bill Inman's original list of Seven Deadly Sins is at this British Medical Association web address:

http://www.bma.org.uk/ap.nsf/Content/AdverseDrugReactions~lowrate

It says among other things:

> "Compared to other countries the number of spontaneous reports submitted in the UK is relatively high and reporting rates in relation to prescription volumes are also among the best in Europe. It is estimated, however, that only 10 per cent of serious reactions and between two and four per cent of non-serious reactions are reported. It should be noted that such a

high level of under-reporting will necessarily lead to bias in the data collected via the Yellow Card Scheme."

Under-reporting, to state the obvious, is bound to lead to bias in the data held by the MHRA—so much so, that one wonders if any statement made by them can ever be regarded as definitive and scientifically valid. In the BMA online discussion, the assertion was made that a recent survey of UK healthcare professionals showed that the only 'sin' still affecting reporting of ADRs was 'lethargy'. This is unlikely to be true but Vivienne Nathanson, head of ethics and science at the BMA, exhorted in July 2004:

> "Doctors must make sure they report any suspected [adverse drug reactions] and at the same time increase awareness among their patients about the reporting process."

So, it has long been known that doctors do not report all the suspected side-effects their patients tell them about. Ten years ago, the BMA issued similar guidance to doctors about the reporting scheme, but it had little noticeable effect. Underlying all is the suspicion that as well as the above reasons, doctors who might report adverse reactions are handicapped by the undoubted fact that the manufacturers have not passed on all they know about the drug. Important too is something which most patients are not aware of—doctors are pragmatists. If one drug fails or is deemed to be inadequate or under-performing, then most doctors will add another in a search for the Holy Grail of a cure. This is, in spite of the fact that all drugs have side-effects, as even pharmaceutical companies themselves now admit—usually when defending the latest drug scandal.

> "People are beginning to say for the first time—if prescribers actually prescribe these drugs, are forced to prescribe these drugs, without all the information that they ought to have, this comes close to fraud."
> Professor David Healy, Evidence to Parliamentary Health Committee, January 2005

So when patients suffer the side-effects of benzodiazepines, prescribed now for nearly 50 years, most of them are not recognised as such, and many, if recognised, are not reported.

In the UK the Yellow Card system and its workings has been clothed in secrecy, based on a belief held by the Regulator that disclosure of detailed figures and decision-making is beyond the ken of ordinary mortals. Dr June Raine, who runs the Yellow Card Scheme for the MHRA, has said on several occasions that she has continually encouraged healthcare professionals to use it. But they do not—and how effective is the system anyway?

In 2003 Dr Andrew Herxheimer and Charles Medawar, were given, as they quite rightly said, unique access to more than a thousand yellow card reports about the SSRI Seroxat/Paxil. Dr Herxheimer is a clinical pharmacologist and was for many years the Editor of the Drug and Therapeutics Bulletin published by the UK Consumers' Association. He works in the international Cochrane Collaboration and is working on a Database of Individual Patient Experience of Illness (DIPEx). Charles Medawar is the Director of health consumer group Social Audit Ltd.

Their analysis found that the nature, the scope and severity of ADRs relating to drug dependency and suicidal behaviour from the antidepressant paroxetine (Paxil/Seroxat) had been concealed and distorted under the present UK reporting system. Their analysis: 'A Comparison of Adverse Drug Reaction Reports from Professionals and Users, Relating to Risk of Dependence and Suicidal Behaviour with Paroxetine [Paxil],' was published in the International Journal of Risk & Safety in Medicine 16 (2003/2004) 5–19. The article was posted at:
http://www.socialaudit.org.uk/5100what.htm#5.1

Dr Herxheimer said that the findings threw into question the value of the existing Yellow Card Scheme, and questioned whether the data produced by the scheme could effectively highlight problems in a time-frame that would protect patients. He described it as "chaotic and misconceived". Charles Medawar and he both said that the information reports are wasted because they are not analysed properly. They argued that their value is limited by the emphasis on numbers not words; the focus on rare and 'interesting' adverse drug reactions, rather than the generality of drug-induced problems. And they pointed to the secrecy that obstructs wider access to anonymised data, and lack of input from users of medicines themselves. On the Social Audit website, Charles Medawar wrote:

> "Our analyses suggest that reports from patients—in their own words—communicate essential information which professional reporters can never be expected to provide."

Without any sense of irony a Department of Health spokesman said, following the findings highlighted in the BBC Panorama programme 'Seroxat: Emails from the Edge', broadcast on 11 May 2003:

> "Patients' views and experiences can make an important contribution."

This was puzzling news to campaigners on benzodiazepines who had been trying to educate the department and its regulators for thirty years or more on the real impact of these drugs on health and lives and the nature of the addiction. The department has stubbornly and frustratingly refused to be educated, and sticks to an approved hymn sheet of words and phrases which interpreted, say that government takes it all extremely seriously and has done (and is doing) everything it can to safeguard and assist patients. But in any case, if you have a problem with prescribed benzodiazepines, then you are on a par with illegal drug users—basically your situation is your own responsibility. How seriously the government takes it is illustrated by the fact that in Professor Ashton's estimate there are still around one hundred and eighty prescribed benzodiazepine addicts per GP practice. The transcript of the Seroxat programme is at:
http://news.bbc.co.uk/nol/shared/spl/hi/programmes/panorama/transcripts/emailsfromtheedge.txt

In its May 2006 report, the British Medical Association said that approximately 250,000 patients are admitted every year to hospital in the UK with adverse reactions to drugs. In repeating its call to health professionals to inform regulators every time an unwanted reaction to a drug is suspected, it was only saying what has been said many times before—that adverse reactions are **"significantly under-reported"**. A 2004 study had found 6.5% of people admitted to hospital had experienced an adverse drug reaction, and that in 80% of these cases the reaction was the cause of the admission. It also found that 2% of patients admitted to hospital with an ADR died. Dr Vivienne Nathanson said after the report:

> "Unfortunately too many health professionals are confused about reporting procedures."

This was confirmed after the MHRA, commissioned the Ipsos MORI poll in 2006. Professor Kent Woods, Chief Executive of the MHRA, said they welcomed the findings and were reassured by the public's confidence in medicines and medical devices. The poll found among other things that over 90% of doctors seemed oblivious to the fact that suspected adverse drug reactions should be reported to the MHRA. No more than one in five doctors was aware that the MHRA regulates medicines and devices. In spite of that, almost 90% of doctors thought that medicines are adequately regulated in the UK. Most worryingly for the patient, doctors saw drugs risk assessment as a trial and error process whereby they 'experiment' with new drugs. It is doubtful whether the many thousands of benzodiazepine-damaged patients were ever aware that they were part of a medical experiment. But as Vivienne Nathanson also said (and others have said it before her):

> "When a drug is first marketed...relatively little may be known about its safety in the population at large."

It is worth adding here that if, as with benzodiazepines, and now with SSRIs, the experiment and denial of damage goes on for long enough, the scale of the harm becomes impossible to admit. Patients, who have suffered injury from drug prescriptions, then suffer a second injury through the concerted establishment denial that the harm occurred in the first place. Unsurprisingly, the political view of SSRIs coming from government is somewhat different:

> "Serious side-effects are rare in the case of Seroxat and SSRIs. Suicidal behaviour during treatment may be linked to illness and may not necessarily be due to the drug."
> Melanie Johnson, Parliamentary Under-Secretary of State for Health, Westminster Debate, 10 November 2004

A flavour of the Yellow Card issue can be garnered from the 2004/5 House of Commons Health Committee Inquiry, 'The Influence of the Pharmaceutical Industry'. There were several keys points and criticisms made to the Committee in January 2005 about the system for adverse reaction reporting and about the MHRA—the DoH Agency responsible for running it.

Professor Healy was not sure that the industry was the real problem however. He said there were two groups he was more worried about—the MHRA, who were not doing their job that well, and the other was physicians generally. The MHRA believe that the Yellow Card system they have is one of the best in the world in terms of trying to track hazards that may be thrown up by drugs in the real world, but Professor Healy went on to say:

> "In actual fact here in the UK we track the fate of parcels through the post one hundred times more accurately than you track the fate of people who have been killed by SSRI or other drugs. If you or your wives or children were to go to your GP and be put on one of these drugs and be injured or killed by these drugs, your GP would not file a Yellow Card with the MHRA. The system as it stands is worthless..."

Richard Brook said that in his view the regulatory system monitoring drug safety, was a secretive affair and he was personally very concerned about it. He recommended that the MHRA be strongly regulated, presumably to ensure that it carries out its stated role in a manner which is ethical, scientific and efficient.

It is hard to have confidence in the transparency of a regulator, when so many of its expert members have a career history in pharmaceutical companies. The current head of MHRA licensing for example had a major role in GlaxoSmithKline regarding worldwide drug safety and the head of enforcement had a twenty year career with GlaxoSmithKline before he became head of enforcement. Brook has said:

> "It seems to me that even in a criminal investigation situation such as, say, the worst case of murder, we actually get more information than we do about how drugs are regulated."

Professor Sir Alasdair Breckenridge, the chairman of the MHRA makes much of the Agency's recent conversion to 'transparency', in a new era of communication. The MHRA has reviewed the Yellow Card system independently and has put on its website all the adverse reactions to every licensed drug to be accessible to everyone, suitably anonymised. But all they really posted were rather outdated aggregate **numbers** of reports—and not the (anonymised) details of individual cases which were needed for research purposes. Professor Kent Woods said:

> "We had an independent external review of our communications activities which reported some months ago—earlier last year and, as a consequence of that, we are forming within the Agency the Communications Division. That will bring together some 26/27 people, many of whom are already in the organisation, but we are drawing this together as a focus of activity. We have appointed a Director of Communications, who will take up post in about ten days' time and we are also investing about £1 million in our website over the next six months..."

Charles Medawar says on the subject of the new system of patient reporting introduced following the damning House of Commons Inquiry:

> "All the evidence suggests to me that the DoH overruled the MHRA and required them to introduce patient reporting as a sop—to soften (or was it enhance) the effect of the Metters [Dr Jeremy Metters, Deputy Chief Medical Officer] review of Yellow Cards. I can remember that even a few days after the announcement was made that Yellow Cards from patients would be welcomed, the MHRA website still had a note saying they were not accepted from patients because medical verification...was essential..."

And given the doubts about the impartiality and efficiency of the MHRA, the fact that you, the patient, can now report adverse reactions, tells you nothing about how seriously or professionally they will be examined and acted upon. You may be less than fully reassured that in future, injuries may be fewer because the regulator has garnered from patients the fact that the drugs do cause injury. As Charles Medawar pointed out—for regulators the question of drug safety revolves around **drug** safety, not the safety of **patients**. It is an important point:

> "The authorities and experts still tend to think in terms of "the safety of medicines" rather than the safety of the people for whom they are prescribed. The powers that be continue to think and act as if safety can be achieved by looking ever more closely at the drug but never too closely at themselves or the system of medicines' control..."
> Charles Medawar, 'Power and Dependence' 1992

And as Professor Andrew Herxheimer, told the Parliamentary Health Committee:

> "I would also like to add that the reports from patients—the MHRA has no idea how to deal with them. I think it would be far better for some other body to deal with those, obviously in connection or consultation with the MHRA, but I have no confidence in the MHRA being able to analyse and understand them."

Professor Breckenridge, after years of criticism of the adverse reaction reporting system, now professes to have seen the light and believes its improvement is vital for the future:

The House of Commons Health Select Committee

> Q852 Dr Taylor: How can you get the medical profession to fill in more Yellow Cards?
> Professor Sir Alasdair Breckenridge: Thank you for asking that question! I hoped you would ask that question because this has come up several times. Dr Taylor, we are very clear in the instructions which we give that we want reports of drugs which have a black triangle and serious adverse reactions. That is what we want. We are very keen to encourage Yellow Card reporting but what we do not want is a lot more reports of rashes on penicillin and bleeding on Warfarin. The Yellow Card system is not there to give an incidence of adverse

> reactions. It cannot do that. It is there to give—and this is a terribly important question that you have asked—a signal where we can take that signal and explore it in other ways. So, while we do want more adverse reaction reports and Yellow Cards, the main thing is that we want better ones and the interesting thing, coming back to what June (Dr Raine) was saying, is that, when we have patient reporting, what kind of profile of adverse reactions will this give us? How will this add to our information on the safety of medicines? That is a very interesting thing which we are going to explore with the new way in which we are doing things."
> Evidence to Parliamentary Health Committee, January 2005

Obviously the MHRA is still exploring and may have lost its way—more than two years after the Select Committee Report they have yet to come up with concrete proposals.

Professor Herxheimer, at the Inquiry, gave an excellent summary about why patient protection will not improve until there is recognition by politicians and the medical establishment that there actually is a problem with the relationship between the MHRA and the Pharmaceutical Industry:

> "I think that the whole basis of medicine regulation started with Thalidomide, and then there was the Sainsbury Committee and the Medicines Act, and that was very much influenced by the industry, what was to be in the Medicines Act, how strong or weak, etcetera. The whole confidentiality, the issue of commercial confidentiality, meant that anything submitted by a company to the regulators could not be disclosed under penalty of fines and prison, etcetera, and that meant that many, many things could be discussed in the regulator, in the regulator agency, which were absolutely private; so that was a very privileged position; that led over the years, over the 40 or more years, to a closeness between the regulators and companies that they were often meeting to discuss details of submissions, information to be given on the package insert and the product characteristics, and so on—they became one community—and so, when the agency was hived off from the Department of Health, became independently funded, independent of government funding, was funded by the industry, the culture became confirmed that the industry is the client and the client must be looked after: quick service, good service, easy contact, etcetera—so it is a closed community in a sense—and outsiders were related to this either by being

appointed to one of the committees of the regulators, the Committee on Safety of Medicines and sub-committees, and thereby tied into the culture of secrecy, signing every document as commercially confidential, or whatever; but commercial confidentiality was never defined, so the anxiety, which has been mentioned already, of the regulators, of the civil servants in the agency, that they might be sued by a company for breach of confidentiality—the Department has a horror of being sued by a company for this, and so there have been very few prosecutions by the agency of companies for various misdemeanours. **All this has led to this close inbred relationship**..." [My emphasis]

And as Professor Ashton said at Bristol in 2005:

"This year the House of Commons Health Committee issued a report entitled "The Influence of the Pharmaceutical Industry". The conclusions were damning. The report states: "The Department of Health has for too long assumed that the interests of health and the [pharmaceutical] industry are one...The crux of the problem is that the Department of Health sponsors both the drug industry and public health matters...**the government's response was to ignore this recommendation."** [My emphasis]

But then the politicians see a different set of priorities. This was the government's concerned comment on the Committee's recommendations:

"The pharmaceutical industry is of enormous importance...to Britain. **It is in all our interests that the industry maintains its currently strong position**." [My emphasis]
Rt. Hon Jane Kennedy MP, Minister of State for Quality and Patient Safety, 2 September 2005

Ministry of Denial

> "The Department of Health...set up an inter-departmental committee to decide on what should be done...This said, and I've seen the report—that it would be very serious if smoking were reduced, because they liked people to die off at 65 to save their pensions."
> Sir Richard Doll, Scientist who proved the link between smoking and cancer.
> Observer/Guardian, April 24 2004

> "The Department of Health fails even to collect figures that might be considered unpalatable."
> Alice Miles, The Times, July 4 2007

Successive governments have allowed tranquilliser damage to continue to blight lives, but the Labour government which took office in 1997 is the first administration to make denial an art form—it is an administration quite prepared to swear black is white.

'Why doesn't the government do something?' Campaigners have heard this plea from benzodiazepine-injured patients and former patients, so many times, they have lost count. They now hear the same thing being said by victims of SSRIs and antipsychotics. It is infinitely depressing to be the victim of a state system and to find no acknowledgement or real concern. It is every bit as bad as being falsely gaoled and finding no route to justice. It is compounded when those who are historically damaged individuals, can see the same thing happening to people all over again with new drugs. It is deeply disturbing to be reminded of how what happened to your life was allowed to happen, and to find that system still in place, with the same score being followed and the notes repeated. Perhaps the aspect with the most impact is an instant recognition of the official refusal to accept and value patient and independent scientific evidence of injury. Benzodiazepine sufferers and campaigners have been met with:

- Blame of the patient based on an establishment philosophy and not on science.
- A pretend policy of meaningful action and a considered refusal to understand that the action is not and never has been, meaningful.

- A policy of deliberate non-understanding of the scale of injury.
- A policy of non-understanding regarding the nature of the injury.
- A capricious refusal to examine the causes of the injury and make changes.
- Self-serving maintenance of an assertion that there is no difference between a person who becomes addicted through illegal use of the drugs and a patient who became dependent because of what his doctor advised and prescribed.

These responses have been—and with variations still are the responses of the Department of Health, in the face of reliable estimates of around one million UK dependent patients.

From time to time, even as a victim of long-term benzodiazepine prescribing and its consequences, you can find yourself reflecting whether it actually **is true** that the Department has done so little that has had a preventative impact. That consideration is not long-lasting, and you return to the question of **why** it has done so little. Benzodiazepines may have been placed in the more user-friendly but totally euphemistic grouping of 'minor tranquillisers', but the range of possible effects is far from minor when prescribed for more than a very short time.

Campaigners, a few MPs and some expert academics—most notably, Professor C.H. Ashton, have attempted to enlighten the DoH on the real world of benzodiazepine injury over very many years, with few measures being taken as a consequence. This says a great deal about how seriously anyone should ever value the rhythmic assertions of the Department of Health, that they take a problem seriously. They did not take health protection seriously with tranquillisers, any more than they take the dangers associated with SSRI antidepressants seriously—at least not as the concept is understood by patients.

Patient safety, it has been shown very clearly—most recently at the Parliamentary Health Committee Inquiry in 2004–5, is not something which the drug regulatory mechanisms in the UK are well equipped to oversee. More than that, the philosophy of those employed to oversee safety, centres around benefit, something which is highly likely to be linked to the revolving door between the pharmaceutical industry and the regulators. Actions which might be taken are restricted by law, which concentrates far too much on the close protection of pharmaceutical company interests. Responsibilities which you might think the regulators should have, such as following up prescribing Guidelines to doctors, they do not apparently have. All these matters ultimately lie within the power to resolve of the Department of Health at Richmond House in London.

If you accept that Ministers of Health **would** do something effective to change the situation if they became convinced of the greater truth of what campaigners were telling them, then it can be argued that the biggest obstacle to improvement has to lie in the political process, which is referred to as the democratic process. I have become convinced that the political system stands between truth and action. It can prevent knowledge being acquired by those who could effect change, and is a dam holding back the introduction of measures to prevent drug damage.

The politician is a generalist and knows little about specifics. Professor Bryan Gould, a former Shadow Cabinet member of the Labour Party, described this fact clearly in 'Goodbye to All That':

> "I knew very little about the subject and was almost entirely dependent on the views of others. Worse than that, I had no means of making a proper judgement as to which view should be preferred. My predicament was common among MPs. Virtually none had enough expertise to enable them to make independent judgements."

The politician then, has no real knowledge of the subject matter of the department for which he is responsible. This fact is exacerbated by the practice of moving ministers around departments at frequent intervals. They are politically responsible for the actions of departments, but are, more than likely, entirely dependent on advisers and civil servants within their department for facts upon which to base political judgements.

Benzodiazepine campaigners are obliged to follow political procedure, as are all who want to inform government and initiate change. If you do not have the contacts or political influence to follow an inside track, there are two possible avenues. For the individual, it involves writing or speaking to the MP of the constituency where you live. That MP, if he feels so inclined, will raise the matter with the minister and ask for comments. The MP will then return the official response to you. Campaigning groups might be able to contact the minister directly. But in both cases, the minister, having no personal knowledge or expertise, will refer the matter to the professionals in the department, who supposedly do have the expertise to deal with it. These in turn will consult official department policy. It is in the area of policy that everything becomes murky.

Policy makers are an anonymous group of people. No one outside the system knows when the policy was made, how it was arrived at, or who made it. You can make an educated guess that benzodiazepine policy was likely to have been made by representatives from the drugs regulator, other experts linked to the pharmaceutical companies, Pharma itself, and the political and financial realists at the Treasury. As someone outside the system, you cannot name them, and cannot comment on the truth and accuracy, or otherwise, of their judgements and arguments. Their formula is what the minister signs. And if the policy flies in the face of what you know to be true, how do you change it? The minister could make changes, but he is far more likely to be influenced by those in the department who see another truth and slavishly follow the results of hidden deliberations. In this scenario, the democratic element in the process, the politician, has no ability to deal with the questions raised, and the undemocratic element, the unelected professional, produces the ministerial reply. The politician legitimises inaction and the avoidance of action.

It is one of the hardest things for victims of medicine to accept, that there is no way they can produce change, without being able to cut through what passes for the democratic process; that those charged with patient safety, like a rubber ball, feel more inclined to bounce off in the other direction towards self protection and denial.

It is clear to an increasing number, that Pharma runs government health policy, both directly and at a distance, through Pharma-captured opinion leaders, regulators and Pharma-financed and on-message medical scientists. These groups are mutually assured, they promote each other into positions of expertise—one influences the other, and they all influence governments from their positions of power. As for what is true—truth is not surprisingly, owned by those with the voice the public hears. The message the public hears is not that of the consumer but the message of the medical establishment—we have the public ear and therefore truth is what we say it is.

There are those however, who find it easier to believe that ministers are not entirely without involvement or significant responsibility. In 1994, two Labour politicians, who subsequently held high office in government after 1997, David Blunkett MP and Paul Boeteng MP, wrote that they understood the scandal of benzodiazepines and would seek to influence government policy and change it. Blunkett became a minister in the Department of Health and was later in charge of the Home Office, responsible for drug classification. Boeteng became a minister in the Treasury. The policy did not change. Denial, semantics and avoidance, continued to be the order of the day.

In October 2003, Professor C.H. Ashton, Jim Dobbin MP, John Grogan MP and campaigners, met Rosie Winterton, the Minister of State for Health. They outlined the impact of benzodiazepines and explained that there was no help available in withdrawal for patients made dependent by doctors. Barry Haslam, a victim of Ativan, who runs a voluntary support group in Oldham and who has campaigned for years, distinctly remembers her looking very surprised and declaring that she had obviously been misinformed. This seemed positive for a while, but when the written reply came from the Department, the traditional position remained unaltered. What had happened after the meeting? Had Rosie Winterton really been surprised? Did she really feel she had been misinformed? If both were true, then this starkly illustrates the power of official policy and those who make it. It would also say something perhaps about the persuasive power of those professionals who surround a minister, mitigating the truth.

Politicians make ridiculous statements on health matters, and the question has to be, are they aware that what they are saying is a rejection of independent evidence and human experience, or are they saying what they do because it serves their own self-interest as politicians and a bigger picture that they believe they see, and victims cannot? On 7 December 1999, in a House of Commons Debate, as the official record Hansard reports, John Hutton MP, the Minister of State at the Department of Health said:

> "My hon. Friend raised the issue of the side-effects of pregnant women using benzodiazepines. I understand and am currently advised, that there is no proven link between benzodiazepine use and damage to developing foetuses."

At around the same time that Hutton was spouting this arrant and dangerous nonsense in Parliament—a statement based as he put it on 'existing evidence'—Dr James Robertson of the Arrowe Park Hospital, Liverpool was saying a different thing:

> "Benzodiazepines cause a more significant withdrawal for the newborn baby than either heroin or methadone...they cry with a cry that is very distinctive."
>
> "...benzo babies will suffer painful cold turkey...and will require intensive care for up to two and a half months...far longer than babies born to mothers addicted to illegal 'hard drugs'."
> BBC Radio 4, 'Face the Facts', March 1999

Two years earlier, Heather Ashton had said that benzodiazepines could affect brain development by stopping the development of natural tranquillisers:

> "There is much evidence to link benzodiazepines with floppy babies and that they suffer withdrawal symptoms. Benzo babies may have similar neurological problems to the babies of alcoholic mothers, such as reflexes which aren't so sharp."

In the same year, the Department of Health's own Committee on Safety of Medicines had issued a reminder to doctors:

BENZODIAZEPINES

Reminder: Avoid benzodiazepines in pregnancy and lactation

Volume 23 (Pages 9–12) September 1997

Benzodiazepines cross the placenta and there is a risk of adverse effects in the foetus. If benzodiazepines are administered at high doses, during late pregnancy, or during labour, effects on the neonate such as hypothermia, hypotonia and moderate respiratory depression, may occur.

Infants born to mothers who take benzodiazepines chronically during the latter stages of pregnancy may develop physical dependence and be at risk of developing withdrawal symptoms (irritability or difficulty with feeding) in the postnatal period.

If a benzodiazepine is prescribed to a woman of childbearing potential, she should be advised to contact her physician regarding discontinuation of the drug if she intends to become, or suspects that she is, pregnant.

Since benzodiazepines are excreted in breast milk, they should not be given to lactating mothers.

From the 1970s onwards, even the manufacturers had warned against using them in pregnancy. The Roche data sheet warned from 1973 that:

> "There is no evidence as to drug safety in human pregnancy, nor is there evidence from animal work that it is free from hazard."

Wyeth's data sheet warned:

> "Safety for use in pregnancy has not been established."

A year after the Hutton statement in November 2000, Keith Hellawell, the government's drugs 'Tsar' of the time, said that he was aware of the problems that women and pregnant drug-misusers faced but then went on to say :

> "The Women's Unit in the Cabinet Office, the Department of Health and the Home Office have been looking at the problems caused by taking prescribed drugs during pregnancy. Consequently, we will be funding the first comprehensive study of services currently available to women, the barriers they face **and identifying the gaps in provision**. Over £1million from the Confiscated Assets Fund will finance this initiative for the next two years."

How much credence should anyone, including MPs, give to anything said by a minister of health in Parliament or anywhere else? At the time when Hutton was summarily disclaiming any departmental knowledge of benzodiazepine harm in pregnancy, doctors in hospital practice knew that it was not true. The Committee on the Safety of Medicines knew it was not true, though as usual, it protected itself by talking about risk and not evidence. Asking doctors to advise women to think about stopping the drug if they were about to become pregnant or were pregnant, was both an inadequate response to the mountain of patient evidence of harm and a very careful avoidance of any examination of the reckless benzodiazepine prescribing practices that had been taking place for nearly 40 years. There would be no follow up to see if the advice—brief though it was, had sunk in—that was not part of the CSM's responsibility. Keith Hellawell was more interested in identifying gaps in service provision for pregnant women than in protecting them and their babies from harm. There was no reference to medical responsibility for prescribing levels that were leading to the damage in the foetus and newborn. This is the way of modern medicine—give subdued warnings when unavoidable, but at all costs avoid saying anything which might be a pointer to blame. If possible stress an old, or even better, a new initiative, which usually impacts little on the problem, but which sounds like serious concern and action.

The Department of Health could have done something to prevent continuing injury to patients, and still could now, but somehow finds itself constrained from action. When the CSM sent out guidance to doctors in 1988 advising them to restrict prescribing to between two and four weeks, it could have acted responsibly and followed it up. It might, without annoying doctors too much (something it always seeks to avoid), have provided finance to undertake a survey of each surgery to ascertain who was being prescribed benzodiazepines, at what level, and for how long they had been taking them. It might, if it had wanted to, have broadened the survey, to ascertain what other drugs each dependent patient had been prescribed. Contrast the no follow-up benzodiazepine situation with the following, reported in the Guardian in June 2007:

> "GPs will be asked to trawl through their patients' records to identify those most at risk of developing cardiovascular disease and call them in for an assessment, the National Institute for Health and Clinical Excellence proposed today."

The Department of Health has never wanted to know anything about the common 'benzodiazepines mean other drugs' phenomenon, and so a large number of doctors have never become aware of it, with the patient as a result, bearing the consequences. Withdrawal from benzodiazepines is not the relatively simple matter the Department maintains and it would rather not know that benzodiazepine addiction routinely exposes people to the possibility of withdrawal from several drugs, therefore forming an even bigger scandal than the DoH already knows exists.

Money is the only thing that focuses the collective mind of the Department. In any discussion of benzodiazepine drug damage, or any other drug damage come to that, the cost to the NHS is the headline figure. The cost to the patient and to society in general is never mentioned. However, the cost to the patient and to society is not just financial—though that is enormous. There is also a wide-ranging and dire negative social impact. In pursuing its line of withdrawal help being readily available and there being no need to set up dedicated financial arrangements, the Department has never quite grasped that prescribers may be efficient at addicting patients but are extremely inefficient at un-addicting them. The DoH steadfastly maintains that a GP can do it, and if not, there are other services available, including psychiatric hospitals, ready to put the patient back on the road to health. The fact that this is simply not true, does not apparently concern them. For the Department, making a statement seems to make it reality. The moral argument never seems to attach itself to ministerial thinking. The patient is given benzodiazepines for a hundred different reasons, becomes addicted, (not unusually losing a job and health), and can then look forward to the caring state providing a place in a psychiatric hospital to get well again. This seems perfectly reasonable to ministers. I have never heard of a psychiatric hospital finding an iatrogenic addict a job, or putting a family back together again, or even being able to deal scientifically with what is in fact chemical dependency injury and not a mental illness.

The Department of Health has always fought against responsibility, and these days it follows what it believes to be Route Number One—pointing to local responsibility. Previously, when it had to, the Department pointed the finger at doctors. Of course prescribers did hold responsibility, though in practice, such responsibility really ends with a prescription signature. The DoH does not wish to appreciate that before the prescription pad comes drug licensing and regulation, and that along with that comes departmental responsibility to formulate a working safe-use-of-drugs policy with a direct responsibility to assist patients who were victims of practices that were not safe.

The following are relatively recent letters which have passed between benzodiazepine campaigners and the Department. It should not take too long to construct an understanding of just how seriously the Department actually takes the 'problem'. The Department of Health and its agencies have recognised for nearly thirty years that the drugs are ineffective in the long-term, and for nearly twenty years have acknowledged that they cause addiction and impact on health. During that period, a way of controlling prescribing, which has continued in spite of 'guidance', has somehow never been found and the victims have never been acknowledged. It is worth noting here, that most letters to the Department are never answered nor receive acknowledgements.

The first of the letters is a written submission to the Department, by Professor C.H. Ashton. It explains that there are still enormous numbers of benzodiazepine patients in the UK. These patients are in theory under the protection of the Department of Health. The submission mentions the move of benzodiazepines into the illegal market. This usually attracts more interest from the department, as it has often demonstrated that it is more concerned with illegal drug use than it is with the same drugs given legally as prescriptions. Official interest was indeed captured, and with the use of cynical spin, the DoH has turned the reality, extending and resurrecting an age-old medical defence argument—centred on the wilful patient. Without coming right out and saying it, the DoH has seized on the illegal factor and now seeks to group iatrogenically-harmed patients with illegal users as part of the same problem. Professor Ashton points to the fact that there are no dedicated withdrawal facilities, and dependent patients are normally referred to facilities designed for people who could be said to have personal responsibility—facilities for alcoholics and illegal hard drug users. Some patients are sent to psychiatric hospitals for rapid withdrawal. But more often that not, patients are not even given this dubious opportunity. Instead their lives are left to wither in their homes, neglected by their doctors, most of whom still have no idea of how to assist patients in withdrawal and have little idea of how bad withdrawal is. If patients are very lucky and live in the right part of the country, they can seek advice from self-financing, volunteer groups. But there are very few such groups in existence. Professor Ashton outlined what she termed 'modest short-term aims for improvement'.

Submission to Department of Health from Professor Heather Ashton, DM, FRCP, October 14 2003
Meeting attended by Rosie Winterton MP, Minister of State, DoH, Phil Woolas MP, John Grogan MP, Jim Dobbin MP

> There are still about one million long-term, prescribed benzodiazepine users in the UK. Our own survey in Newcastle found an average of 186 such patients in every GP practice. Similar figures have been obtained in surveys in Gateshead, Liverpool and other UK general practices.

These patients, taking prescribed benzodiazepines regularly for six months, a year, often many years, have become dependent on the drugs through no fault of their own, yet they receive little medical help or advice. Almost daily I receive letters, phone calls and emails from such people who claim that they get scant support from their doctors and almost none if they wish to withdraw their medication.
In fact benzodiazepines are still affecting people at all stages of life, from the elderly who take them chronically as sleeping pills or are given them to keep them quiet in retirement homes, to young and middle-aged patients still being prescribed potent benzodiazepines such as Ativan for long periods, to psychiatric patients discharged into the community, still taking benzodiazepines started in hospital, to women being prescribed during pregnancy and thus their developing foetuses and newborn infants. And finally this over prescription has led to benzodiazepines leaking into the illicit drug scene—there are about a hundred thousand so-called "recreational" benzodiazepine abusers in the UK who take the drugs illegally (with all the health and social risks of polydrug abuse, including hepatitis and HIV), and this number is growing rapidly.

I ran an NHS benzodiazepine withdrawal clinic in Newcastle for 12 years from 1982–1994. The success rate for withdrawal was nearly 90% and the patients' physical and mental health improved. But when I retired, this clinic closed, along with other dedicated NHS withdrawal clinics throughout the UK. As far as I know, there are none left now. Some benzodiazepine dependent subjects have been diverted to "detox" units designed for alcoholics and users of hard drugs, but such clinics are highly unsuitable for benzodiazepine patients. Other patients are simply left to fend for themselves or to attend charities and self-help groups which receive little public funding.

It is a well-established fact that long-term benzodiazepine use leads to physical and mental health problems. In addition there were 1810 deaths from benzodiazepine overdose 1990–1996 according to Home Office Statistics and there are an estimated 1600 benzodiazepine-related traffic accidents with 110 deaths each year in the UK.
There is a regrettable paucity of available treatments for such patients. This is partly because many doctors have not heeded

the advice of the Committee on Safety of Medicines, circulated to all doctors in 1988, that prescriptions should be short-term only two to four weeks, and that benzodiazepines should not be prescribed to patients with depression, and partly because doctors are unsure how to handle benzodiazepine withdrawal, despite the sound advice available in the British National Formulary that all doctors receive.
The only contributions I have been able to make since having by law to retire from NHS practice at the age of 65 is to write the booklet "Benzodiazepines How they work and How to Withdraw" (available free on the Internet), to give advice to local support groups and charities such as the North East Council for Addictions (NECA) in Newcastle, and to answer several hundreds of personal requests for advice.

I submit that there are some minimum immediate requirements for action that the Government could and should take now:
a) The CSM should issue repeat guidelines on benzodiazepine prescription and withdrawal methods to all doctors, and the Chief Medical Officer should also issue a statement to all doctors outlining the problem and providing guidelines for prescription and withdrawal. I would be happy to assist in the drafting of such documents.
b) The Government should provide finance for health workers, such as community nurses and pharmacists and counsellors, to attend GP practices to support patients withdrawing from benzodiazepines. They can supply the much needed regular patient contact that GPs don't have sufficient time for. This approach has already proved successful in some centres but needs to be extended nationwide.
c) The Government should provide grants to support groups such as Council for Involuntary Tranquilliser Addiction (CITA), Bristol & District Tranquilliser Project, North East Council for Addictions (NECA), the Oldham Group and others to set up and run benzodiazepine support and withdrawal centres. Many of these groups have more knowledge and experience of benzodiazepine problems than doctors.
These are modest short-term aims. Long-term, research and development of non-drug treatments for anxiety and insomnia is needed, as well as better education of doctors on long-term drug effects. Already there are problems arising with non-benzodiazepine hypnotics such as the "Z-drugs" (zopiclone, zolpidem and zaleplon) which are being prescribed instead of

> benzodiazepines but are causing the same problems including dependence and abuse.
>
> It is a tragedy that these steps are needed 50 years after benzodiazepines were first introduced. They could have been foreseen and prevented but instead the skeleton was locked in the cupboard for many years. Now we are faced with worms that are crawling out of the woodwork including not only the problems of long-term prescribed users but also the increasing spectre of illicit benzodiazepine abuse.
>
> C.H. Ashton

For an appreciation of the official mind, the reply from Rosie Winterton gives the government response to the request for what most people would regard as the very least that the innocent were due. This second letter is one more marvel of Health Department production:

> Thank you for a very helpful meeting in October to discuss the issues associated with benzodiazepine prescribing and the problems experienced by those who are now dependent. Thank you also for the documents you have supplied.
>
> First of all let me say that the Department of Health, the NHS and the various professional groups regard involuntary addiction upon benzodiazepine drugs as a very important issue. We have taken a number of steps to tackle the problem, and we are encouraged that the number of prescriptions is now falling.
>
> As you know, the main focus of the Department of Health's action in this area has been to try and prevent addiction/dependence occurring in the first place by warning GPs and other prescribers of the potential side-effects of prescribed medicines and the dangers of involuntary addiction.
>
> I know you are aware of the advice issued in the British National Formulary (BNF), updated twice yearly and issued free to all doctors, and the advice issued by the Committee on Safety of Medicines (CSM).
>
> In addition, we have commissioned the National Institute of Clinical Excellence to develop a guideline on the management of anxiety. This will include recommendations about drug treatments. I believe we can remind GPs of how important this is by publishing a short note in the Chief Medical Officer's Update and I will ensure that this is done.
>
> At the meeting, the dangers of illicit drug taking and of the operation of a black market in tranquillisers, was mentioned. I understand that a common means of obtaining diverted drugs

is by deception of the general practitioners either through plausible exaggerations of daily consumption or multiple registrations with different GPs, commonly as a temporary resident.

As you know, responsibility for prescribing, including the issue of repeat prescribing of tranquillisers, rests with the doctor who has an ethical responsibility to inform patients about the treatment proposed, including any possible side-effects of prescribed medicines. It is the responsibility of the PCT to ensure that adequate controls of prescribing are in place. Conspicuous poor prescribing would result in disciplinary action, either from the PCT or from the General Medical Council. The use of clinical audit and peer review has also provided a powerful incentive for local clinicians to study their patterns of care and improve prescribing standards.

It is the responsibility of the prescribing doctor to try to ensure that any drugs issued are not diverted onto the illicit market. The Misuse of Drugs Act 1971 makes it illegal to supply benzodiazepines to someone else. Provisions contained in the Criminal Justice Bill that comes into force on 29th January this year mean that the maximum penalty will be changed from 5 years in prison and a fine to 14 years. I understand you have concerns about how to change the controls in place relating to these drugs. Of course this is a matter for the Home Office, but I suspect the more promising approach for people who suffer dependence is to ensure there is good awareness among patients, the public and the NHS, and an adequate range of services.

For those who have developed dependence upon tranquillisers, treatment is available in primary and/or secondary care settings. Anxiety management, which may be on an individual or group basis, often includes some focus on reduction or cessation of tranquillisers. Such therapy may be available in Clinical Psychology Departments, via a Day Hospital or from a Community Health Team.

I realize that waiting lists for 'talking treatments' can sometimes be too long. This is why we set out standards for access to treatment in the National Service Framework for mental health and issued guidance to help GPs and service users and carers know more about the effective treatments in 2001. Copies of this guidance are available at:
www.doh.gov.uk/mentalhealth.

I acknowledge the point made that advice and guidance on prevention is not always enough, but we have to work with the levers that are available to us. This is why, to strengthen the performance management arrangements in place to support best practice, we recently asked the Commission for Health Improvement (CHI) to consider including waiting times for psychological therapies as one of the Performance indicators for mental health trusts, which is still under discussion.

In addition to this, since our meeting, there has been extensive discussion with CHI about the PCT Performance indicators relating to prescribing. Although I understand you may be disappointed at the outcome, we were persuaded by the arguments made by the CHI and others that we should not restrict our attention to the Benzodiazepine group of drugs alone. We have therefore agreed to broaden the focus and extend this PI to include other drugs such as antidepressants and anti-psychotics as well. Information about this has been placed recently on the CHI website www.chi.nhs.uk.

Last but by no means least I would urge you to contact the National Institute for Mental Health's (NIMHE) Expert by Experience Programme. I would like to see better information available for benzodiazepine users about the scope for supported self help, and about best practice. (NIMHE) is supporting dissemination of information for service users and carers and I believe there may be an opportunity for you to strengthen this.

I am copying this letter to Jim Dobbin MP and Phil Woolas MP and I assume you will share this letter with those who accompanied you to the meeting.

Rosie Winterton MP, Minister of State, Department of Health, January 11 2004

That the medical and political world takes the problem seriously is the message, twenty or thirty years after it first took the matter seriously. It has taken it so seriously that it has looked on while doctors have continued to make patients dependent on dangerous drugs. It is clear that the medical profession is an entity which is not to be curbed or tackled head-on in the light of official knowledge of damage to patients. Medicine is a unique profession, which is to be addressed politely, without too much alarming detail of the nature and extent of the damage it causes.

Professor Ashton replied to the minister regarding her sanguine use of statistics, pointing to a fall in benzodiazepine prescriptions. As she says, this is largely due to the vast increase in prescriptions for SSRI antidepressants, and the rise of 'Z' drugs, the effects of which are the subject of another struggle by patients, academics and campaigning groups. With her experience, she cannily spotted the attempt by the

Department to side-step the real issue by talking about legal penalties applying to patients passing on prescriptions. As she said, helping patients to stop taking the prescriptions in the first place would be more to the point.

The Minister did not address the position of the formerly dependent patients who now found themselves apparently permanently damaged, but then why would the Department want to do that? There was no money forthcoming for withdrawal services, so ensuring assistance for the permanently disabled, would be seen as even more of a step too far. This step too far should never be undertaken, in case of wider repercussions and discussion around the purpose of medicine and the effectiveness of drug regulation.

> Dear Ms. Winterton,
> Thank you for your letter about the meeting with John Grogan and others last October 14th, which has now been passed on to me. We appreciate your having given thought to many of the points we raised about involuntary dependence on prescribed benzodiazepines. However, I would like to raise some further issues.
>
> (1) You say in your letter that you are encouraged that the number of prescriptions for benzodiazepines is now falling. Unfortunately, as we pointed out at the meeting, this fall is largely due to prescriptions being shifted to the "Z-drugs" (zopiclone, zolpidem and zaleplon) which have all the same disadvantages of the benzodiazepines including drug dependence (addiction) and are more expensive.
> There were 3.57 million prescriptions for these drugs in England in 2001–2 and 3.99 million in 2002–3 (Prescription Pricing Authority—PPP). The National Institute for Clinical Excellence (NICE) is looking into these "Z-drugs" at present and is not likely to recommend them over benzodiazepines, indicating that, unless steps are taken, benzodiazepine prescriptions are likely to rise again.
> Some of the fall in benzodiazepine prescriptions is also due to a shift towards antidepressants which are more toxic than benzodiazepines and also produce withdrawal ("discontinuation") effects. Thus the fall in benzodiazepine prescriptions does not necessarily signify a benefit to patients and is not necessarily a basis for encouragement.
>
> (2) We are aware of the excellent advice about benzodiazepines in the British National Formulary (BNF) and that of the Committee on Safety of Medicines (CSM).

Unfortunately, doctors are not heeding this advice and, as I mentioned at the meeting, surveys in Newcastle, Gateshead, Sunderland, Liverpool and other parts of the country show that there are on average over 180 long-term (6 months to many years) prescribed benzodiazepine users in every general practice despite the guidelines that prescriptions should be limited to 2–4 weeks only. Prescribing is no higher in the North of England than elsewhere and there are over 1 million long-term prescribed benzodiazepine users in the UK.

For this reason, we welcome your assurance that the Chief Medical Officer will publish a "short note" (though why is "short" specified?) to remind GPs with advice on benzodiazepine prescribing, and that you have commissioned NICE to develop a guideline on the management of anxiety.

(3) However, the management of anxiety, though it may possibly help to limit future anxiolytic benzodiazepine prescriptions, does not address the root of the problem that we hoped to draw to your attention at the meeting. It should not be assumed that all benzodiazepines are prescribed for anxiety. In fact almost twice as many benzodiazepines are prescribed as hypnotics. In 2002–3 there were 5.67 million prescriptions for benzodiazepine anxiolytics in England but 10.45 million for benzodiazepine hypnotics (PPP). In addition, many benzodiazepines were prescribed for conditions unrelated to anxiety e.g. as muscle relaxants in orthopaedics, for post-flu depression, menstrual problems and home difficulties (Ashton 1987). Many of these people have become benzodiazepine-dependent after prolonged use.

What is needed are dedicated clinics or other arrangements to help people already dependent on benzodiazepines to withdraw. You state that "treatment is available in primary and/or secondary care settings" for those who have developed dependence on tranquillisers. This is simply not the case. I and many others in the field get daily telephone calls/letters/e-mails from benzodiazepine-dependent people who are desperate because they are receiving no help or advice from their doctors and cannot find any support groups or benzodiazepine withdrawal clinics. I also mentioned this point at the meeting.

"Talking treatments" by psychologists, for which you rightly say there are long waiting times, are not always appropriate for benzodiazepine-dependent patients. Clinical psychologists are very rarely aware of the special problems, withdrawal effects, or withdrawal methods for benzodiazepine users. Anxiety management is not always indicated for users of benzodiazepine hypnotics or anxiolytics. The patients need specific information about benzodiazepine-related problems including withdrawal symptoms and personalised withdrawal schedules. Such expertise is usually not in the remit, training or experience of clinical psychologists, as I know from my own experience in my benzodiazepine withdrawal clinic. (Addiction clinics for alcohol and illicit drug abuse are clearly inappropriate for these patients.).

Much more beneficial would be the setting up of support groups in the community dedicated to benzodiazepine-dependent clients. These could be staffed by counsellors who are ex-benzodiazepine users trained by a similar scheme which has been set up for ex-heroin users to become drug counsellors. In addition, the participation of trained community nurses, community pharmacists and counsellors in GP surgeries should be encouraged. This approach has already worked well in some areas including Liverpool (as mentioned by Pam Armstrong at the meeting) and Newcastle where the North East Council for Addictions (NECA) and community pharmacists have provided counsellors and pharmacists to GP surgeries. Perhaps the CMO could write not only to doctors but also to pharmacists' and nurses' organisations to encourage this approach.

(4) You mention that the maximum penalty for supply of benzodiazepines to the illicit market will be increased from 5–14 years in prison and a fine. At the meeting, it was pointed out that much of these supplies come from elderly ladies on repeat prescriptions of the hypnotic temazepam (who have taken them for years) who pass on all or part of their prescriptions to their younger relatives. Imprisoning little old ladies will hardly solve this problem! Helping these elderly ladies to stop taking benzodiazepines would be much more to the point and is sometimes feasible with minimal intervention (Heather et al. 2004; Cormack et al. 1994; Bashir et al. 1994). Other users may require more prolonged, experienced and dedicated support in support groups and GP surgeries as detailed above.

(5) There is no mention in your letter, or in the minutes, of the plight of many ex-benzodiazepine users who have been left with apparently permanent cognitive and physical damage as

a result of long-term prescribed benzodiazepine use. This problem was cogently illustrated at our meeting by a carer of such a patient. Many of these people have difficulty in obtaining DSS benefits because their disability is not recognised. Prolonged and sometimes irreversible sequelae of chronic, often high dose, prescribed benzodiazepine use has been well documented (Ashton 1995). This point should be mentioned in the CMO's "short note" and sent to the DSS so that those affected receive more sympathetic treatment.

(6) I regret to say that the minutes fail to record many of the issues discussed at our meeting. Some of the points may therefore be missed if the minutes are viewed as the "official record". However, a list of follow-up actions is mentioned at the end of the minutes. We have received no feedback on some of these and are not clear whether the suggested actions have been taken.

(7) Finally, we are, as you expected, "disappointed by the outcome" of our meeting, especially for the lack of financial help to set up dedicated benzodiazepine withdrawal clinics. We note that you feel constrained by "the levers that are available" to you, but surely it is the Department of Health that should lead in pressing those levers. For your information, a meeting has been arranged in Bristol on February 4th 2004 with the European Commissioner for Health and Consumer Protection, Mr. David Byrne, and reports on UK and European drug issues, written by Barry Haslam, will be handed over at the meeting.
C.H. Ashton, 26 January 2004

I wrote this letter on 7 February 2004 to the minister to give further input to the argument. It remained unacknowledged.

Dear Ms Winterton,
In recent days you referred to your awareness of the 'problem of benzodiazepines'. But I wonder if that is really so. Such 'awareness' has been stated and restated by ministers since the 1980s, and benzodiazepine over-prescribing is still with us. References to the total number of prescriptions falling is hardly evidence of a concerted effort to tackle the wrongful prescribing of a group of drugs which can destroy health and life generally, without bringing more than a few days or weeks of benefit to any patient.

The drugs are not recommended for use beyond four weeks for good reasons. Even before that time, for some patients, physiological and psychological dependence/addiction occurs. All addictions are harmful, and some infinitely more than others. Benzodiazepines can rightly be said to be the "damned when you take them, and damned when you stop" drugs for many. Their effect on the mind and body during, and often long after addiction, is so severe that the NHS spends large amounts of money continually conducting tests for apparently 'real' illnesses, when in fact the sole problem is the drug. The effect on the unaware patient is of course more personal and immediate. In addition doctors have been allowed to believe that outward side-effects of the addiction such as self harm, aggression, increased anxiety and depression are symptomatic of further illness, when in fact these things are clearly related to the drugs. This belief usually results in the 'topping up' of benzos with other drugs—often SSRIs, tricyclics and hypnotics, which are themselves toxic and merely deepen the trap caused by the primary addiction.
No one knows (including the Department of Health) how many lives have been destroyed by the over-prescription of the benzodiazepine class of drugs, most particularly since 1988, but we believe that the Liberal Democrat MEP Chris Davies described the situation fairly when he said recently that,

"Because those affected don't have to steal to fund their habit, but instead get the drugs from the health service, their plight goes largely unnoticed by society. But the social cost of family breakdowns and individual impairment is immense."

Journalist and former MP, Matthew Parris, may have had part of the picture too when he said in an ITV programme on 29 January, after revisiting the Scotswood area of Newcastle,

"I was stunned...at the sea of Prozac on which this entire locality seems to be afloat...so many people seem to be on Prozac. At first I felt angry that doctors should prescribe it so easily...People are being drugged here by the National Health Service to quieten them down, and parents are conniving in this and drugging their own children—diagnosing their own children with Attention Deficit Syndrome...The British state is just drugging people into submission because they are less of a nuisance that way."

It is hard for any observer, looking at the history of the years since Librium was licensed without proper scientific trials, to gain any sense of determination on the part of the health authorities in this country to do anything effective about the 'problem', thereby promoting a view that government actually prefers this situation. Referring to available levers is a rather Pontius Pilate-like argument, and I am sure the officials who advise you are completely aware of that. Any government which took the health of the population seriously—and we are told by the Secretary of State that yours does, would solve the 'problem' with the creation of new 'levers'. Keeping your eye fixed on the scarcity of prescribing doctors and the perceived need for doctors to be able to prescribe something for the realities experienced in deprived areas and for the problems of life generally, is perpetuating drug harm on a scale well above that of illegal drugs.

Every reference by government and in the media to the impact on health of drugs like ecstasy and heroin is a painful reminder to former patients that politics is not about morality but about pragmatism and avoidance of responsibility. It is because prescribed mind drug harm is not 'sexy' and the media is transient in its attention to it, that successive governments have been able to allow the destruction of lives to continue, while promoting the welfare of the pharmaceutical industry. The population too, by the basic facts of human nature, is willing to believe that if they are ill they will receive beneficial treatment and that a doctor knows what he's doing when he prescribes drugs. This ensures a perpetual supply of drug victims, and as numbers mount, so avoidance of responsibility for the past becomes increasingly important.

The word expert in medicine has become one of the most self-serving terms in the language. Experts such as Professor John Marks come, are willingly believed, do their damage, and move on. The 'non-experts' pay the price. Drug companies know well the value society places on the word 'expert'. As part of their strategy for profit, they actively foster the careers of believers, and the believers foster the strategy for profit. Most of the membership of the MHRA/CSM is politically naive and incestuous, but at the moment the regulatory system in place is the only protection the population has. Its former incarnation, the CRM, believed that benzodiazepine addiction was almost impossible. It had its mind changed by public pressure, issued Guidelines in 1988, but apparently it has no basic remit to follow up its own recommendations.

Responsibility has been so diffused in the Health service that it amounts as far as benzodiazepine prescribing is concerned, to no responsibility. Any complaint by a patient about drug harm leads to a door being closed and a finger pointed to another. Doctors have an ethical responsibility? In practice the responsibility of a doctor ends with the prescription pad, and ethics is largely a question of historical philosophy. Most doctors are a hybrid mixture of good intentions, mixed in with a large degree of pragmatism, naivety and ignorance. The ignorance of the effects of drugs is the central factor in prescription drug harm and it is maintained by the ability the ABPI and individual drug companies have, to block, control, and interpret information reaching doctors. There is too the lack of any real sense of urgency or explanation in the information available through Prodigy, NICE and the BNF. Moreover the freedom of a doctor to ignore advice (unlike teachers who are regulated in the minutiae of teaching) is crucial. It has been nearly fifty years since benzodiazepine damage began, a small sense of urgency would seem appropriate.

Government may believe that informing doctors of what they **should** do in respect of prescribing, and then leaving the rest to PCTs and prescribers is government responsibility fulfilled, but in a state-funded health service—a social enterprise, someone should have prime responsibility for ensuring that health recommendations actually happen. No one has it in the present set-up, and certainly not government, apparently. Patients pay the price for this.

The fact that most points to your non-understanding of the 'problem', is contained in your statement that help for benzodiazepine addiction is available in Primary/Secondary care settings. In theory this may be so, but in practice the view is completely at variance with experience. Dedicated clinics that did exist have closed, for reasons of finance, not because the need was markedly less. Even Hazel Blears' infamous statement about help for those addicted to prescription drugs being available in Drug Misuse centres was not at all accurate. Clinical Psychologist appointments are extremely difficult to obtain and since anxiety is typically short-term, cognitive therapy is hardly likely to have much of an impact if seen as an alternative to drugs, in view of the time scale involved and the chronic shortage of psychologists and therapists. Talking therapies after addiction are not likely to have too much impact either, since the anxiety the psychologist would be likely to see would be chemically produced.

No one addicted to benzodiazepines has a chance to improve their lives, caught up as they are in the side-effects. These and drug tolerance (cravings for more of the same to produce equilibrium) frequently occasion a constant malaise. If drug treatment is to be the mainstay of NHS treatment, the very least you can do as a health department is institute proper regulation which constantly reviews drug effects in reality, rather than in theory. A system which, when it does decide to issue advice to doctors, has the remit to follow up advice is needed. Better still would be an independent system outside the Department of Health, which seems to be quite hopelessly confused by its dual functions of health and promotion of the pharmaceutical industry.

Fifteen years of doctor education, albeit low key, has failed to stop the harm. A better policy and new 'lever' might well be to educate the public in prescription drug safety as the Belgian government intends to do. Ethical responsibilities, for many doctors, do not seem not to extend to putting patients in the picture when a drug is prescribed, partly because they are not aware of the full picture themselves. Packet warnings about addiction on benzodiazepines would be a good start. It is hard to see how the ABPI could object to this, since after decades of maintaining that the drugs were non-addictive, data sheets have acknowledged it since 1999. Individual patients might be at least prompted to be on their guard about what they are taking and be able to ask their doctor why the warning is there.

There is now no winnable scientific argument about whether benzodiazepines are addictive—even the most dyed-in-the-wool advocate, one who doesn't understand human chemistry and prefers to blame the patient, admits to a 30% addiction rate. It is more than a pity that the Department of Health, rather than protect the citizens of the UK from drug harm, prefers to play with words, to point to responsibilities which are largely avoided, and give a picture of progress based on a raw reduction in numbers of prescriptions. The reduction is not due

> much to improvements in prescribing, but rather to a shift towards other toxic substances such as SSRIs and the 'Z' drugs such as Zopiclone—the latter apparently coming under grave suspicion in Ireland and becoming a problem for NICE.
>
> Benzodiazepines cure nothing. They are intended to be, as the WHO has said, a medical short-term palliative. The status of the drugs as 'essential drugs', is not based on the way they are prescribed in the real world, but on the way they should be prescribed. Benzodiazepines cure nothing but they inflict much harm in the long-term. The Department of Health should stop pretending that over-prescription is a medical judgement. Over-prescription is a gross and extremely damaging medical misjudgement. Benzodiazepines, for the addicted, replace one temporary illness or problem with a large number of new ones, often coming after the drug is stopped, if it ever is. Those in the Department who have convinced themselves that only bona fide psychiatric cases are given benzodiazepines, thereby justifying manufacturer claims that symptoms often return when the drug is stopped, should consult the many and varied reasons for prescription.
> Colin Downes-Grainger, Benzodiazepine Campaigner

The Chief Medical Officer did indeed send a communication to all doctors and as Professor Ashton pointed out to the Minister, some doctors took this to mean that dependent patients should be immediately withdrawn, leading to further injury. As an indication of the seriousness of the situation, the most central point the CMO could come up with, was the financial cost to the NHS, which as I suggested earlier, is very far from accurate, given the propensity of benzodiazepines to lead to other prescriptions, most of them being far more costly than the cause of those prescriptions. And naturally there was no mention of the cost to patients, financial or otherwise. It often seems to me that if medicine had an additional remit – say social work, it would know far more about risk/benefit than it does now. Note the assertion that there are 'specialist clinics' in 'some parts of the country' dealing with benzodiazepine dependence. No mention of where they were, or what their 'specialist' nature was.

But the most brazen (and galling to patients) proposal, to deal with a situation created by doctors, was the proposed plan to introduce instalment prescribing. What was at the core of that intention? The central meaning seems clear. This situation is not one any doctor need feel responsibility for—let the patient deal with the consequences. It is the patient who has wilfully insisted on continuing to take the prescriptions on which they have become dependent, so doling them out is an appropriate measure.

Benzodiazepines Warning from the Chief Medical Officer, January 2004

Doctors are being reminded that benzodiazepines should only be prescribed for short-term treatment, in light of continued reports about problems with long-term use.

Clear Guidance for appropriate use was published in 1988 by the Committee on Safety in Medicines (CSM) (sic*)*, which recommended Benzodiazepine should be prescribed for: just two to four weeks for relief of severe or disabling anxiety that is subjecting the patient to unacceptable distress; and severe or disabling insomnia in patients who are extremely distressed.

They should not be prescribed for the treatment of mild anxiety, according to the CSM. Although prescribing of benzodiazepines has declined substantially since the release of CSM advice in 1988, prescribing has continued for patients with insomnia and anxiety and for substance misusers.

Department of Health data show that in 2002, 30% of prescriptions for benzodiazepines were for 56 or more tablets (see box), which suggests a high number of patients are receiving long-term treatment. Long-term use exposes patients to risks such as road traffic accidents, dependence and, in the older population, debilitating falls.

Reducing use

Echoing the CSM advice, the Mental Health National Service Framework (NSF), which was published in 1999, recommended that benzodiazepines should be used for no more than two to four weeks for severe and disabling anxiety.

The Mental Health NSF called upon health authorities to implement systems for monitoring and reviewing prescribing of benzodiazepines within local clinical audit programmes. Primary Care Trusts (PCTs) should ensure that this recommendation is still being implemented.

Experts say consistency in approach and effective communication between primary and secondary care health professionals could help reduce over-prescribing. Such communication could involve the use of shared treatment guidelines that specify duration of therapy and cessation of treatment following hospital discharge.

More attention should be paid to the prescribing of benzodiazepines for older people. This could possibly be achieved during the regular medication reviews entitled to all people over 65, according to the Older People's National Service Framework.

Use of benzodiazepines in substance misusers is still an area of concern. It is estimated that 14% of substance misusers attending drug treatment centres report benzodiazepine use subsidiary to their main drug use.

Benzodiazepines by the numbers

General Practitioners in England wrote 12.7m prescriptions at a cost of £20.9m in 2002, compared to 15.8m prescriptions worth £13.8m in 1992. (Newer agents are more expensive, leading to higher costs despite a drop in prescription volume.)
30% of prescriptions were for 56 or more tablets.
People over 65 years received 56% of prescriptions for the three most commonly prescribed benzodiazepines.
Source: Department of Health, 2002 data, England

The Department of Health is planning to introduce instalment dispensing of benzodiazepines to minimise access to excessive doses for addicted patients. Also, in some parts of the country, specialist clinics are available to help people with benzodiazepine dependence.

For more information on appropriate prescribing, see:
British National Formulary, guidance on management of benzodiazepine dependence.
DoH Drug Misuse and Dependence, Guidelines on Clinical Management, 1999 .
MeReC Briefing, Issue No.17, April 2002, update on benzodiazepines and non-benzodiazepine hypnotics.
Prodigy, hypnotic and anxiolytic dependence and insomnia.
The Clinical Governance Research and Development Unit at the University of Leicester, audit protocol and data collection forms for prescribing in primary care.
Department of Health contact is Gul Root, Richmond House, 79 Whitehall, SW1A 2NL. Email: gul.root@doh.gsi.gov.uk

Since Gul Root was given as the contact in the CMO's update, Barry Haslam, benzodiazepine campaigner and volunteer consultant, wrote to that worthy at the Department, regarding the value of instalment prescribing for iatrogenic addicts and for information regarding the CMO's assertion regarding specialist clinics. The reply was as follows:

> Dear Mr Haslam
> In your letter you have asked for a list of specialist clinics for patients who are dependent on benzodiazepines. As you are probably aware, Professor C.H. Ashton ran a dedicated benzodiazepine clinic in the Newcastle area for about twelve years, which helped many patients withdraw from benzodiazepines successfully. We are aware that some Primary Care Trusts have developed schemes to reduce prescribing of benzodiazepines. For example, St Helen's PCT has developed a benzodiazepine resource pack for all GPs. Pharmacists also visit GP practices providing one to one sessions to advise on withdrawal strategies for appropriate patients. The services of a benzodiazepine counsellor who is based in the local Walk-in-Centre are promoted during these sessions. The PCT also plan to set up a user group drawing on the experience of people who have successfully withdrawn from benzodiazepines to help those who are on treatment currently to withdraw.
>
> The Department of Health funded Medicine Management Collaborative, which is being rolled out in waves, has demonstrated innovation and good practice in many aspects of medicines management. Currently there are four waves in operation covering 146 PCTs and with around 14,000 GPs and 4,900 community pharmacies. When these schemes are fully rolled out across these PCTs there is the potential for over 27 million of the population to be getting help to make better use of their medicines.
>
> There are currently at least 7 PCTs within the Collaborative programme who have developed schemes to improve benzodiazepine prescribing. For example, East Birmingham PCT has developed guidelines and a toolkit for anxiolytic and hypnotic prescribing. The guidelines incorporate withdrawal strategies that can be used by GPs. The PCT is also planning to set up pharmacist-led clinics in the near future to help patients withdraw from treatment where appropriate. Other initiatives include a scheme for the management of benzodiazepine/hypnotic withdrawal at Hartlepool PCT, development of a benzodiazepine resource and audit pack at

Huddersfield Central PCT, Information to support benzodiazepine audit at Wakefield PCT.
An addiction therapist who works across the two Wakefield PCTs helps and supports patients, especially those over 55 years of age, identified by the audit as having been on benzodiazepines on a long-term basis, to withdraw from treatment. Many patients seen by the therapist have withdrawn from treatment all together. More details about the schemes can be obtained from Richard Seal, Director of Medicines Management at the National Prescribing Centre.
We hope to implement instalment dispensing of benzodiazepines for the management of addiction over the next year and are currently exploring regulatory and other changes required to make it possible. I am not able to provide any further details about the scheme at this moment of time.

Instalment 'dispensing' allows a single prescription to be written for a patient whilst allowing the pharmacist to dispense the medicine to the patients over a number of days. This avoids the need for a separate prescription for each instalment dispensed, making it simpler for a prescriber to limit the amount of medicine a patient has dispensed in one go. This also has benefits for the patient as they do not have to go to the GP each time they need their medicine dispensed. This will be particularly useful for addicted patients on benzodiazepines who may be liable to misuse their medicine.
Gul Root, Principal Pharmaceutical Officer, Public Health and Community Services, Department of Health, 13 May 2004

There is the clearest indication yet in the next letter, that the Department has little concern for patients or for a medical scandal that it has watched happening. The Department recognised that patients might feel there was a stigma attached to being seen as having a mental health problem when in fact it was entirely a chemical problem, acquired through prescriptions from doctors. But nevertheless, the establishment of specialist benzodiazepine dependence treatment services was not seen as cost effective or an efficient use of resources. Not cost effective? But the Chief Medical Officer had said they existed—at least in some parts of the country, hadn't he?

Dear Mr Haslam
Thank you for your letter of 24 June to John Reid concerning Benzodiazepine (sic). As you will appreciate, Mr Reid receives large amounts of correspondence and cannot answer all this

mail personally. Your letter has been passed to me and I hope that you will find the following reply helpful.

We would like to reassure those with dependence on benzodiazepines that many people access services in and through primary care, including people whose main problem is physical rather than psychological or psychiatric. Such arrangements help to ensure a multidisciplinary approach and that the widest range of knowledge and capability can be brought to bear on presenting problems, regardless of their cause. We know that there are concerns about the potential stigma of being treated alongside those with mental health problems that are seen as self-inflicted. However, we do not believe that establishing specialist benzodiazepine dependence treatment services would be a cost effective or efficient use of resources.

User and carer involvement is nowhere more important than it is in mental health. Empowering patients to take an active role in their care is a key theme in the Government's mental health policy. This is why prescribers should inform patients about the treatment proposed, including any possible side-effects of prescribed medicines.

K. Horner, Customer Service Centre, Department of Health, 13 July 2004

What is cost effective? In 2005, the northern town of Oldham, which has a scheme dedicated to benzodiazepine withdrawal, spent £44,424. It reportedly helped 15 people in that year. Oldham has an estimated 5000 or so dependent patients. With around one million such people nationally, anyone with a calculator can do the maths. I calculate that in Oldham, if there were no new dependent patients added to the list and the assistance was universally successful, then funding of £16 or £17 million would be required. Nationally that would mean multiplying the figure two hundred times. That figure would not include the costs of training specialists to undertake the task and the costs of setting up a system of training. These costs would necessarily apply since the Department refuses to allow that ex-patients are the true experts on withdrawal, and there are a great many such ex-patients available.

Perhaps the cost is what the Department understands by cost effective. But beyond that, policy makers and/or succeeding politicians, may be more concerned about the political cost attached to a demonstration of how intractable the problem is, how long-standing it is and how it was allowed to develop. Barry Haslam replied as follows:

> Thank you for your letter dated 13th July 2004. I have the following comments to make:
>
> **1**. You stated that those dependent on Benzodiazepines can access services in and through Primary Care.
>
> Question: Please will you send me full details of those services provided through Primary Care and which Trusts offer such a service?
>
> 2. You admit that dependence on Benzodiazepines is a physical one, i.e. a Chemical Addiction.
>
> Question: Why then is the Psychiatric Unit used as the sole means of withdrawing Benzo addicts, when they have a physical problem, not a mental health problem?
>
> 3. You state "However, we do not believe that establishing specialist benzodiazepine Dependence Treatment Services would be a cost effective or efficient use of resources."
>
> Questions:
>
> a. Can you tell me who the "we" are in your above statement- i.e. person or persons responsible for this decision?
>
> b. Can you let me have detailed costings to prove your argument of "not cost-effective or efficient use of resources."?
>
> c. What other comparative addiction treatment services did you equate Benzodiazepines with?
>
> d. Can you give me the date when the decision was taken not to establish specialist Benzodiazepine Treatment Services?
>
> 4. With 1.2 million people currently addicted (long-term) to Benzodiazepine drugs in the UK, your letter of 13th July, 2004, is crass, insulting, and shows a basic lack of knowledge of Benzodiazepine drugs and their dangerous consequences.
>
> 5. Services for Iatrogenic Addiction should be made a priority for funding by Government, not swept under the carpet. Benzo addicts have become an embarrassment and a liability to the Department of Health, and the medical profession—therefore deny them services, their human rights, and hope the problem will go away! The establishment cover up on benzodiazepine addiction goes on and on.
>
> Barry Haslam, 19th August 2004

In the reply that came back from Kierran Horner, there was a notable withdrawal from what the Department obviously felt may have been an admission too far:

> I am sorry for the delay in replying and I hope that you will find the following information helpful.

> The line from my previous response, “We would like to reassure those with dependence on benzodiazepines that many people access services in and through primary care, including people whose main problem is physical rather than psychological or psychiatric.”, does not imply that the Department believes dependence on benzodiazepines is solely physical.
> As I explain in the next sentence, we aim to ensure people with mental health problems receive the care and treatment they need as individuals and arrangements that help to assure a multidisciplinary approach and ensure the widest range of knowledge and capability can be brought to bear on presenting problems, regardless of their cause, are most beneficial to people with benzodiazepine addiction.
> The Department have no plans to issue central guidance on which forms of benzodiazepine treatment centres are to be provided, and in line with the Department’s policy of Shifting the Balance of Power, decisions about service provision should be taken locally. It is for Primary Care Trusts (PCTs), in conjunction with Strategic Health Authority (SHAs) to plan and develop services according to the needs of their local communities. When commissioning services, PCTs will need to take into account whether it is in line with locally agreed health priorities and that its provision will be a clinical and cost effective use of resources. This does often mean that PCTs have to make difficult decisions about how their finite resource is spent.
> The Department of Health does not hold details of service provision across the country. Your SHA [Strategic Health Authority] may be able to advise if they can provide you with further information about the local services available but as with any other condition, access to specialised services is through a GP and that is where people should refer themselves for assessment. I hope this clarifies the position.
> Kierran Horner, Department of Health, 13 September 2004

The Department delights in repeating back to you things you already know, while avoiding reference to the concerns and realities you actually raised. The pre-formulated letters at the Department brook no amendment. After a letter from me on the subject of Kierran Horner’s reply, I received the following letter from Poonam Bassi. Examine these statements:

> “The main focus of the Department of Health’s action...has been to try to prevent addiction/dependence occurring in the

> first place by warning GPs and other prescribers of the potential side-effects of prescribed medicines..."
> "Conspicuous poor prescribing would result in disciplinary action either from the PCT or from the GMC..."

In respect of the first statement, as usual there is no mention of warning the patient. Health providers do not consider adequate warnings given directly to patients, without mediation, to be necessary, desirable, or part of their remit. This philosophy has led to many ruined lives over the years and is a necessary dovetail for the denial of drug injury. The second assertion is probably false and reflects theory rather than practice. In any case, due to the secrecy involved in medicine, who would ever know?

> Thank you for your letter of 24 September to Kierran Horner at the Department of Health concerning problems in relation to benzodiazepine medication. Your letter has been passed to me and I hope you will find the following reply helpful.
> Benzodiazepine drugs are most commonly prescribed as tranquillisers (for anxiety) and as hypnotics (for insomnia). This group of drugs has been available since the early 1960s. Even at that time it was realised that dependence could develop with high dosage usage but normal dose dependence was not recognised until some time later.
> The product information and articles in the publication Current Problems in Pharmacovigilance warn prescribers that use of benzodiazepines, even at therapeutic doses, may lead to the development of physical dependence. The risk of dependence increases with the dose and the duration of treatment. It is also greater in patients with a history of alcohol and drug abuse or patients with marked personality disorders. Abrupt discontinuation of the therapy may lead to withdrawal or rebound phenomena. Some people suffer symptoms over prolonged periods.
> The Department of Health, the NHS and the various professional groups regard such involuntary addiction as a very important issue and have taken a number of steps to tackle the problem. The main focus of the Department of Health's action in this area has been to try to prevent addiction/dependence occurring in the first place by warning GPs and other prescribers of the potential side-effects of prescribed medicines and the dangers of involuntary addiction to benzodiazepines.
> In 1994, the Department of Health issued copies of Guidelines for the Prevention and Treatment of Benzodiazepine

Dependence published by the Mental Health Foundation, to all Health Authorities and recommended their use by GPs. The Department issued another publication in 1999 entitled Drug Misuse and Dependence—Guidelines on Clinical Management (1999), which reiterates these messages. The British National Formulary (BNF), updated twice yearly and issued free to all doctors is also an important source of guidance on the management of benzodiazepine dependence.

The National Institute for Clinical Excellence (NICE) has started work on the development of a clinical guideline on the management of anxiety. This will cover both drug and non-drug (psychological) treatment approaches and will no doubt consider the use of anxiolytics such as the benzodiazepines.

The Committee on Safety of Medicines (CSM) has issued this advice:

"Benzodiazepines are indicated for the short-term (2–4 weeks) relief of anxiety that is severe, disabling or subjecting the individual to unacceptable distress, occurring alone or in association with insomnia or short-term psychosomatic, organic or psychotic illness.

The use of benzodiazepines to treat short-term (mild) anxiety is inappropriate and unsuitable.

Benzodiazepines should be used to treat insomnia only when it is severe, disabling or subjecting the individual to unacceptable distress."

This advice has led to an overall reduction in the prescribing of these drugs and the attendant dependence problems.

The responsibility for prescribing, including the repeat prescribing of tranquillisers, rests with the doctor or prescriber who has clinical responsibility for that particular aspect of a patient's care. Doctors have an ethical responsibility to inform patients about the treatment proposed, including any possible side-effects of prescribed medicines. It is the responsibility of the Primary Care Trust (PCT) to ensure that adequate controls of prescribing are in place. Conspicuous poor prescribing would result in disciplinary action either from the PCT or from the General Medical Council. The use of clinical audit and peer review has also provided a powerful incentive for local clinicians to study their patterns of care and improve prescribing standards.

More recently, as announced in the Chief Medical Officer's 2004 Update, work is in progress to introduce instalment dispensing to minimise access to high doses. It is planned that this will be in place in 2005.

The emphasis is thus mainly on preventing such addiction from occurring in the first place, but for those who have developed dependence on tranquillisers, treatment may be offered in primary and/or secondary care settings. Anxiety management, which may be on an individual or group basis often includes some focus on reduction or cessation of tranquillisers. Such therapy in secondary care may be available in Clinical Psychology Departments, via a Day Hospital or from a Community Mental Health Team.

The work I mentioned above being conducted by NICE will serve to emphasise the evidence behind these approaches. The Mental Health National Service Framework and the NHS Plan, which has mental health as one of its clinical priority areas indicate that there needs to be a focus on evidence-based psychological and other treatments, including drug, treatments for mental health problems. Expansions within mental health service provision would not just be for those with psychotic illness and provided by specialist services but also there would be extra provision within primary care mental health.

I hope this information is helpful in responding to your concerns.

Poonam Bassi, Customer Service Centre, Department of Health, October 2004

Michael Meacher, a former cabinet minister who has shown consistent concern about the impact of benzodiazepines on his constituents wrote to Rosie Winterton on the subject. Note again, in the reply, the capricious assertion by the Department about where responsibility lies for iatrogenic dependence. Though a Department spokesman later made a kind of withdrawal, referring to 'mis-wording,' the attitude has never been clearer.

Thank you for your letter of 10 November enclosing correspondence from your constituent Mr Barry Haslam about benzodiazepine addiction.

Decisions on the commissioning of health related services in a community, including those that treat drug misusers, are best made by local stakeholders who are best placed to commission services based on the needs of their local population.

As is the case for those people who misuse drugs, such as heroin and cocaine, we would expect those who misuse benzodiazepines to have access to a range of services both in the primary and secondary care settings to meet their needs.

Your constituent may be aware that drug treatment services, which expanded rapidly in the last few years, have been developed in a way that allows them to meet the needs of the drug misuser, irrespective of their addiction, rather than by developing drug specific services. Figures on numbers accessing and being retained in these services are all positive, which indicates this type of approach does meet the needs of individual drug misusers.

In terms of benzodiazepines, you will be aware that to minimise the risk of overdose and other negative effects of abuse of these drugs, we have changed the general medical service (GMS) regulations to allow for instalment dispensing of these drugs.

I hope Mr Haslam finds this reply helpful.

Rosie Winterton, Health Minister, 14th December 2006

Bridget Prentice MP wrote to Rosie Winterton on behalf of one of her constituents. Again the assertion regarding responsibility was made in the reply, the constituent was, in the eyes of the Department of Health, a drug misuser—end of story. We already knew that the Department 'took the problem seriously' and now we were told that the government was committed to access to services for the problem. What was 'the problem' in official eyes? **The nature of 'the problem' put simply, was one of drug misuse by patients, and their self-motivated addiction to prescriptions.** On the other hand, doing something was a local health authority responsibility, so if you find yourself without access to the services the DoH persistently maintains do exist, you should kindly address your concerns to your Primary Care Trust. Worried that doctors were routinely ignoring DoH guidelines? That was without doubt a PCT responsibility too. Prescriptions had fallen, instalment dispensing was being introduced, and the Chief Medical Officer had sent out an Update. Everything was covered.

Thank you for your letter of 15 November on behalf of your constituent Ms T. regarding benzodiazepine addiction.

I would like to reassure Ms T. that the Government is committed to ensuring that those people who misuse drugs of any kind have access to services that best meet their needs.

In terms of the commissioning of services available within individual areas, this is the responsibility of the NHS at local level, which is able to commission services based on the needs of the local population.

Turning to the points identified in the advertisement enclosed with Ms T.'s letter, I should emphasise that individuals with dependence on benzodiazepines are already able to access a range of services in primary and secondary care. In primary care, counselling, advice and/or psychological therapy are available. Secondary care services are also available, including specialised mental health services and specialised drug services. NHS services are commonly provided on the basis of clinical need rather than the causes of need, and support for benzodiazepine withdrawal can be provided in a range of settings.

On the issue of enforcing guidelines regarding the prescription and usage of drugs by GPs and psychiatrists, there is already clear guidance available. Any practice outside of this guidance should be brought to the attention of the relevant Primary Care Trust with immediate effect. The Committee on Safety of Medicines (CSM) continues to issue advice regarding the prescription of benzodiazepines, emphasising that they should be used for the short-term relief (2–4 weeks) of severe or disabling anxiety, and not for the treatment of mild anxiety. This advice was reiterated in the Chief Medical Officer's Update in 2004. Given concerns about previous over-prescribing, it is of note that the number of benzodiazepine prescriptions issued in England in 2005 fell to under 12 million per annum.

We have also introduced a new 'instalment dispensing' facility, for prescribing diazepam in cases of dependence, which enables these to be dispensed by daily or by less frequent instalment. It enables prescribing professionals to use this mechanism to increase the safety of such prescribing should it be necessary. Prior to this being introduced, prescribers had to write multiple short-term prescriptions to achieve this. The facility had already been available for a number of other controlled drugs for use in the management of dependence for some time prior to its introduction for diazepam.

In terms of updating warnings, this matter is kept constantly under review and, should we conclude that further action needs to be taken in this area, we will not hesitate to do so.

I hope Ms T. finds this reply helpful.

Caroline Flint, Public Health Minister, 18 December 2006

Professor C.H. Ashton wrote to both Ms T. and to Rosie Winterton, having been distinctly underwhelmed by Caroline Flint's assurances.

Dear Ms T.
Thank you for your letter and enclosure.
I see that Caroline Flint rolls out the same old story we have heard again and again from the Department of Health—that individuals dependent on benzodiazepines "are already able to access a range of services in primary and secondary health care". I have pointed out repeatedly to Rosie Winterton and others that this statement is not true.
In primary care the waiting list for "counselling, advice and/or psychological therapy" is up to two years, by which time it is too late for the long-term patient to benefit from it, especially since the therapists are ignorant about the effects of benzodiazepines and withdrawal. Secondary health care services are usually not available for prescribed benzodiazepine users; they are regularly turned down because they are not also using opiates or other "hard drugs". Mental health centres and specialised drug services are in any case inappropriate, and often disastrous, for prescribed benzodiazepine users who are a quite different population from illicit drug users. The "instalment dispensing facility" is a gross insult to prescribed users and reflects the hard-headed ignorance of the Department of Health who seem to be concerned only with illicit drug abusers.
Caroline Flint's letter reveals again that the interests of long-term prescribed users are being fobbed off as usual with weasel words that are not relevant to their case.
The side-effects of zolpidem, zopiclone, zaleplon and eszopiclone are the same as those of benzodiazepines, as recognised by the National Institute of Clinical Excellence (NICE).
I enclose a reply to my letter to Rosie Winterton from one of her deputies, and my response. It seems we are up against a brick wall!
Professor C.H. Ashton, 29 January 2007

Rosie Winterton found herself too busy to reply personally. Instead the Professor received a reply from the 'Customer Service Centre'.

Dear Ms Ashton
Thank you for your letter of 9 January to Rosie Winterton about the prescribing of benzodiazepines. Due to her pressing schedule, it is not always possible for Ms

Winterton to answer all the correspondence she receives personally. I have been asked to reply.

The Government is seeking to reduce waiting times for talking therapies through its Improving Access to Psychological Therapies (IAPT) programme, which began in May 2006. This policy was set out in the Government's 2005 manifesto and in the Our Health, Our Care, Our Say, White Paper. Ministers are looking to develop a service model for delivering a range of evidence-based interventions, with the focus being on cognitive behavioural therapy because this has the broadest evidence base.

Initially, IAPT consists of two national demonstration sites in Newham and Doncaster and a national programme of local projects in each of the National Institute for Mental Health in England's eight regional development centres (RDCs). Ministers aim to work with the RDCs in preparing other areas around England to begin a phased roll-out of service models. It is envisaged that between ten to twenty new services will roll-out in the first wave, on a region-by-region basis, with sites chosen by the strategic health authorities in discussion with their Primary Care Trusts in due course.

Ministers expect IAPT to provide robust evidence in favour of increasing psychological therapy capacity and this will help to clarify the numbers of staff, the skills set and the training requirements needed to do this. A business case will be submitted to Treasury as part of the comprehensive spending review in early 2007, which will make the case for investing in local psychological therapies services across England.

Jane Spencer, Department of Health, 19 January 2007

Professor Ashton replied on 29 January 2007.

Dear Ms Spencer

Thank you for the letter you wrote on behalf of Rosie Winterton. The government's aim to reduce waiting times for talking therapies, especially cognitive behavioural therapy (CBT) may be laudable for patients with depression, but it is clear that neither you nor Rosie Winterton understand the issues with regard to long-term benzodiazepines users. As previously explained, talking therapies, especially CBT, are not helpful for long-term benzodiazepine users who are still taking the drugs because benzodiazepines impair the ability to

> use cognitive strategies as well as impairing judgement and memory.
> The first step is to withdraw these patients from the drugs. This requires support of a different kind as I have previously explained at length and will not reiterate here. So quicker access to talking therapies may prevent long-term use of benzodiazepines for new patients but will be of little value to the million long-term prescribed users in the UK—however many “waves” you "roll-out" on a “region-to-region basis."

It does not matter who says what to the DoH, the reaction stays the same. If correspondence to the Department says something which the Department does not want to hear, the points are simply ignored. In idle moments you wonder how DoH personnel—people with supposed intelligence imagine that the nonsensical gibberish they send out would make even fractional sense to any reader. I often wonder, whether anyone at the department ever stops to think much about who is writing to them and why. Do they ever have a sense of realisation concerning what campaigners are telling them—that patients' lives have been destroyed for nearly half a century, and enough is enough? I think they do, but lack the motivation or ability to empathise too greatly. And not knowing too much about reality is seen as best practice by politicians in power.

The Department has set up a Customer Service Centre, but has it any idea what it is for? Is it more a case of window-dressing to suit the times? What should its purpose be? If you create a Customer Service Centre, presumably you expect the customer to tell you how they feel about the service. A business which consistently, and for so many years, deliberately misunderstood and avoided addressing customer complaints would not stay in business for long. But then the DoH has a captive clientele and in commerce there are customer protections which actually do afford some safeguards in a range of areas. For one thing, the customer has access to law over serious breaches of trust—this is not so with drug damage.

Neither the Customer Services title nor never-ending statements have made patient protection any more real or effective and have certainly not proved that the DoH is listening to a word patients say. Any independent arbiter on the benzodiazepine issue, faced with the evidence and reading the correspondence involved, would find it quite unnecessary to deliberate for long—the conclusion of state indifference in an era of health exploitation is inescapable.

Mendacious Government

"I voted for Labour in 1997 and was very excited about the prospects of them coming into power, but perhaps I was naive. I honestly believed that MPs were bound to care about social justice, decency and morality but I have met so many who don't seem to care. There are not enough MPs who are willing to stand up to ministers who they believe have acted wrongly."
Dr Ros Altmann, former government pensions adviser, Daily Telegraph, February 5 2007

"It seems that, these days, everyone and everything has got a Tsar...over time, of course, the meaning of "Tsar" has changed: originally it meant "emperor", which later blurred to "king". In British politics, it now appears to mean 'damage limitation exercise'. Just as problems within health care have been made public, so the number of Tsars has proliferated... But the problem with being a Tsar is that, while you are there to promote the interests of a group, you are, essentially, on the government payroll...Tsars aren't independent and they're not elected...A Tsar doesn't represent the people; he represents the interests of the Government. We've got more Tsars than the Romanovs, and yet nothing seems to happen..."
Dr Max Pemberton, Daily Telegraph, February 5 2007

"This has been a bad year for mental health [2006]...As the year rolled on, evidence piled up that, despite one in four people in the UK suffering mental ill health at some point in their lifetime, the services that treat them have been disproportionately affected by cuts. Adding insult to injury, the government has refused point blank to accept that this is the case...The minister in charge, Rosie Winterton, responded: "There is no evidence to suggest that mental health services are being disproportionately affected by the current funding situation.""
The Guardian, December 20 2006

"As the government became aware of the disaster it had created...a top priority of [the Department of Health] was to hush it up by ensuring that no minister or official ever publicly

admitted that organo-phosphorus pesticides could cause chronic damage [to the farmers who used them]. This was not only because using the chemicals had been made compulsory, but because each product had been licensed as safe to use by the government's own veterinary medicines directorate."
Private Eye Magazine, 2003

"In early 1987, just after the Thatcher government decided on MMR as an option in mass vaccinations, doctors in America had already reported "adverse reactions" to Urabe MMR. A few months later, the Swedes reported 52 cases of "febrile convulsions probably associated with MMR vaccination"...It took until 1992 for Britain to stop injecting children with Urabe MMR, replacing it with MMR2, which contains a less potent form of the mumps virus. And, according to the minutes, that action owed more to the decision of the manufacturers of Urabe MMR to cease production. Revoking the licence would have cast light on Whitehall's decision to use Urabe MMR on British children despite disturbing evidence of its potential effects."
Daily Telegraph, March 5 2007

"Barbiturate consumption doubled during the 1950s and continued to rise well into the next decade. In 1964, an editorial on the Barbiturate Problem in 'The Practitioner' asked if "this fantastic amount" of barbiturates was really necessary. Questions to this effect were also asked in Parliament, but the Minister of Health was not moved: "I have no evidence that harmful effects or dependence occur at all frequently in relation to the number of prescriptions." Later, and perhaps with some irony, Sir Derrick Dunlop said he thought that such ill-effects were "remarkably rare in Britain considering the prodigal amounts that are prescribed." Sir Derrick was the first head of the Committee on Safety of Drugs, forerunner of the Committee on Safety of Medicines."
Charles Medawar, 'Power and Dependence', 1992

"An independent public inquiry into how thousands of haemophiliacs contracted HIV or hepatitis C from contaminated blood has discovered that Downing Street is withholding crucial information about how hundreds of relevant documents were shredded on two separate occasions between 1990 and 1998. More than 1,700 patients died and

> many more are now terminally ill. Some of the destroyed documents detailed meetings between the blood transfusion service, health boards, government officials and consultants during the Seventies and Eighties. The records also contained information on when precisely the government became aware of the risks from imported blood and what measures were taken to warn patients."
> The Observer, May 2007

The National Health Service became a reality on 5 July 1948 and was the political construct of the Labour party and the then Health Secretary, Aneurin Bevan. Because it is a government creation and is directed through central financial arrangements from Whitehall, it has been routinely defended by politicians from negative experiences and patient complaints.

Bevan brought reluctant hospital consultants on board the newly created NHS by giving them an extremely beneficial contract, where in effect they were independent, were paid a salary by the state but were also allowed to work within the private sector. In Bevan's words he "stuffed their mouths with gold". The treasury refused to finance the incorporation of GP practices into the NHS and so the GPs, working within the state system, were now to be employed as independent contractors, running their own businesses, but receiving a salary from the state. GPs are still independent contractors today—sixty years after the NHS began, and a significant number still top up their state incomes through private work. This is a surreal situation, where the state trains doctors and employs them, but at the same time allows them to work outside the system using an economic model which should apply only to those who do not work for external employers. This situation has caused problems persistently throughout the years. The most damaging result for the victims of prescription drugs has been the continuance of a mindset in government which sees doctors as a unique body of men and women, who must be treated with kid gloves, to be encouraged rather than instructed. This reality can clearly be seen in the following example. In 'The Tranquilliser Trap', Professor Louis Appleby, still today the government's Mental Health Tsar, talked about the central guidelines to doctors on their prescribing of tranquillisers, issued in 1988. He said:

> "I think the guidelines are completely clear. I don't think there's any problem in understanding them. I think what the problem has been that changing individual prescribing practice requires more than guidelines."

But what was it that the government intended to do beyond guidelines? Since the government had no coherent idea how many people were taking tranquillisers long-term, the programme conducted its own survey which showed that the advice had been falling on deaf ears. The guidelines had said prescriptions should not exceed four weeks but Panorama had found that 28% of patients had been taking the drugs for more than ten years. It should be remembered that this was thirteen years after the advice was sent to doctors.

In a letter to former minister Michael Meacher in January 2007, Health Minister, Rosie Winterton said:

> "It is also of note that the number of benzodiazepine prescriptions issued in England has fallen from 14.027 million in 1995 to 11.252 million in 2005."

The government now has some data available, but the central message is studiously not being assimilated. There is in existence a raw number count, but it has no depth, and remains depersonalised. In 2004, following representations from benzodiazepine campaigners, the Chief Medical Officer had written to doctors saying that prescription levels were still too high. Apart from the fact that there seemed to be emphasis only on the cost to the NHS of inappropriate prescribing, the real point—that many doctors still believe their own clinical judgement trumps drug safety warnings, is totally ignored. Government still has no precise idea about prescription levels or the length of those prescriptions for individuals. Responsibility, if there is any, has been put at arm's length and according to the Department of Health, is now the province of local Primary Care Trusts. Government permitted over-prescribing to continue, even when it knew such prescribing was dangerous. Government then devolved responsibility for monitoring it and declared that if there was a problem it should be examined at a local level. It did not see the necessity to put in place a precise system of checks to ascertain whether local oversight was actually taking place.

The primary motivating factor for the UK government is money—the maximisation of income and the minimisation of what it deems to be unnecessary expenditure. Limiting government outgoings is necessarily bound up with the avoidance of responsibility and the rejection of independent evidence based on fact. The history of the benzodiazepine drugs in the UK is the definitive example of the attitudes of government to the issue of prescription drug safety. It has been a story of wilful institutional misunderstanding, sanctioned drug-company misinformation and disinformation, lack of science and since the 1970s, a deliberate and calculated cover-up by Department of Health officials and politicians. To add insult to injury, the department has for years, allowed the continuance of insidious damage to the lives of unaware patients, so that the past will remain unaddressed, calls for compensation will be avoided, and the establishment healthcare system can continue as before. Official silence, rejection of patient evidence, ineffective actions, fingers-crossed references to the 'problem being taken seriously', and manipulation of the media, have all been tactics designed to head off serious examination of the UK drugs regulatory system, with its pervasive pharmaceutical company links. These tactics have also prevented real examination of the role of politicians who persistently maintain that the system is effective, able to assess benefit/risk accurately, and that patients are protected.

For 25 years since the CRM statement in March 1980, the Department of Health has declined to do anything of note to protect the health and lives of patients who could potentially become addicted to prescribed tranquillisers and hypnotics, or who were already addicted to benzodiazepine drugs. No rational explanation has ever been given for the inaction. No Guideline can ever be seen as an effective protection for patients. The NICE website has this to say about Guidelines:

> "Clinical guidelines are recommendations by NICE on the appropriate treatment and care of people with specific diseases and conditions within the NHS. They are based on the best available evidence. **Guidelines help health professionals in their work, but they do not replace their knowledge and skills**." [My emphasis]

In spite of the health damage that has occurred in this country, the best that Ministers and civil servants can do is make statements which are designed to reassure the uninvolved and uninformed that something effective has been done:

> "We regard dependence on benzodiazepines as a very important issue and the Department of Health has taken a number of measures to tackle the problem. The main focus of the Department's action in this area has been to try and prevent addiction from occurring in the first place by warning GPs and other prescribers of the potential side-effects of the prescribed medicines and the dangers of involuntary addiction to benzodiazepines."
> Caroline Adams, Political Office, 10 Downing Street, March 19 2002.

> "We take the problem seriously."
> Anna Higgitt, Senior Policy Adviser, Department of Health, 2002

"...innovation is being rolled out in waves..."
Gul Root, Department of Health, 2004

"...treatment is available in primary and secondary settings..."
Rosie Winterton MP, Department of Health Minister, 2004

In May 2001 Professor Louis Appleby had referred to the benzo situation as a disaster but thereafter he did nothing to ameliorate it. He may have been well aware when he made the statement, that any examination of the logic of the situation from the point of view of affected patients, or the impartial would conclude that it was entirely indefensible. There are still doctors who do not appear to know that tranquillisers cause much ill health and the DoH countenances that ignorance. References to the responsibility of PCTs or the ethical responsibility of doctors is not action, they are merely sound bites. Protection of health is something quite different.

When he was asked on the BBC's 'The Tranquilliser Trap' why nothing had been done to prevent the damage produced by tranquilliser/hypnotics, it is worth wondering whether he had ever stopped to consider the full implications of what he was saying when he said that it was difficult to change the prescribing habits of doctors. At the core of that statement was the strange idea that even if the DoH is aware of the negative health impact of a licensed drug it has no ability to protect citizens from the causes of it.

No doubt patients will find complaints written to the DoH about SSRIs being responded to with formulated non-concern in the same way that letters on benzodiazepines have been replied to. The response will refer to the National Institute for Clinical Excellence advice, the views of the Medicines and Healthcare products Regulatory Authority, the advice in the British National Formulary, the responsibility of the Primary Care Trusts to monitor prescribing and the ethical responsibilities of doctors. And in the meantime the patient must bear full responsibility for side-effects for the simple reason that he or she made the mistake of turning up at a surgery in the first place. That patient will not be recognised by politicians, the General Medical Council, Primary Care Trusts, the drugs regulator, the legal system, or the doctor.

Professor Malcolm Lader said many years ago now, that benzodiazepines were harder to withdraw from than heroin, and harmful effects could go on indefinitely. That being so, patients deserve something more from government than statements which are untrue and mere spin. They merit real support, which actually exists. And for medically created addicts it is particularly galling to see the millions poured into illegal drug addiction support.

Dr Anna Higgitt, once a colleague of Professor Lader, and now the Senior Adviser at the DoH on benzodiazepines, said in 1990:

> "There is no doubt at all that benzodiazepine addiction and its health consequences are an iatrogenic illness and PWS (post withdrawal syndrome) is likely to be a genuine iatrogenic complication of long-term benzodiazepine treatment."

No real improvement has occurred since she gained her position. Is it surprising that the benzo-affected doubt the motives of the Department of Health? The Department of Health apparently does not care and apparently believes it has no responsibility to care. Shifting the balance of power, in the dictionary of government, should more appropriately be described as the creation of a central avoidance strategy. And the final insult, in a scenario where SHAs and PCTs do not provide services, is government insistence that the thousands of medically afflicted should be left to their own limited devices.

Attempts to inform the politicians and officials of the Department of Health about the world of benzodiazepine addiction meets with surreal statements such as the following:

> "User and carer involvement is nowhere more important than it is in mental health. Empowering patients to take an active role in their care is a key theme in the Government's mental health policy. This is why prescribers should inform patients about the treatment proposed, including any possible side-effects of prescribed medicines."

If only patients did hold power. If only prescribers did inform them. If patients had been empowered and had been informed, campaigners would not continue to write to the DoH to report on continuing harm. If the protection of patients from injury was seen as at the centre of healthcare, the creation of new iatrogenic addicts would have ceased long ago.

The government promotes the view that existing arrangements are based on a wide expertise in the field of benzodiazepine addiction and withdrawal. The Department is consistently at pains too, to confine any examination of the tranquilliser question to the psychiatric/psychological field and ignore the essentially physical dimension of the addiction. Mike Shooter said in the BMJ in 2003 that psychiatry was not expert in the area of prescription drug withdrawal. In 2004 the BMA said that GPs did not like dealing with addicts and had little knowledge of withdrawal procedures. I wonder if government appreciates or is concerned by these glaringly obvious contradictions to its statements.

Take benzodiazepines legally and you become a non-person, take them illegally and you become a government concern.

On 13 May 2004, Gul Root, Principal Pharmaceutical Officer, Public Health and Community Services, Department of Health, searching for something which could cast a positive light on the inaction of the Department, gave as assurance that something was being done, a reference to the withdrawal clinic that Professor Ashton ran in Newcastle. Unfortunately for addicted patients, that has not operated since her retirement from the NHS several years ago. One has to wonder why it was mentioned at all, particularly as Professor Ashton is highly critical of department policy. Other seemingly worthy initiatives were described:

> "We are aware that some PCTs have developed schemes to reduce prescribing of benzodiazepines..."

In that respect, in a letter to Barry Haslam of Beat the Benzos in November 2005, Alan Higgins, the Oldham Director of Public Health had this to say:

> "...Oldham PCT is one of a small number of PCTs to not only take the matter of benzodiazepine addiction seriously but to commit resources towards its reduction..."

So after nearly half a century of benzodiazepine mis-prescribing, half a century of medically-induced ill health and half a century of aborted lives and deaths, a small number of local health authorities take the 'problem' of benzodiazepines seriously and the Department of Health maintains the comforting myth that much has been done and is being done—that the responsibility lies at local level. Another interesting statement was:

> "There are currently at least 7 PCTs within the Collaborative programme who have developed schemes to improve benzodiazepine prescribing...When these schemes are fully rolled out across these PCTs there is the potential for over 27 million of the population to be getting help to make better use of their medicines..."

There were 302 PCTs in the country!

If politicians in the Department of Health and government drug regulators had acted years ago in a fashion befitting their stated aims i.e. the safeguarding of public health, instead of preferring to maintain the myth of clinical judgement and the economic vibrancy of pharmaceutical companies, patients would have been able then to make 'better use of their medicines'. But this is not an issue of patients making better use of medicine, this is an issue of a government department playing with words for decades, spinning around the huge damage uninformed doctors had inflicted and still are inflicting with tranquilliser and hypnotic prescriptions.

> "An addiction therapist who works across the two Wakefield PCTs, helps and supports patients, especially those over fifty five years of age, identified by the audit as having been taking benzodiazepines on a long-term basis, to withdraw from treatment..."

Many patients have been on these drugs for anything up to forty-plus years. One therapist to support thousands of patients is really quite breathtaking. This is progress in the eyes of government. This is effective action as far as they are concerned. Gul Root seemed to feel no sense of irony in sending out this message. Apparently it was something to feel pleased about. And who is supporting those whose addiction has ended but whose drug-induced disabilities now rule their lives? The answer to that is certainly not government. The fact that many are disabled after long-term addiction is something that the DoH does not want to acknowledge or think about. Neither does the Department of Work and Pensions, but perhaps the two departments have made a pact that if neither thinks about it or acknowledges it, then the disabilities will dissipate to become in essence non-disabilities. And if officialdom at the centre, or indeed the drug companies, do not recognise a symptom or disability then doctors certainly will not recognise it either. Professor Heather Ashton is not of course the only medical expert to have discovered benzodiazepine disability but so far, judging by its actions, the Health department has not. She said at the Bristol AGM in October 2005:

> "I don't think the powers that be have any idea of what goes on in the lives of individuals, who through failures of the present system, are driven outside the system to seek advice from poorly funded support groups and organisations like this one."

The present Minister of State for Local Government, Phil Woolas, has declared on several occasions that he is convinced that the whole tragedy of benzodiazepines has been deliberately swept under the carpet by government and at a benzodiazepine conference in Oldham in 2004 he went further. He said then that he believed there was an 'organised government cover-up' of the last four and a half decades. Campaigners are fully aware of the truth of this, meeting as they do with consistent indifference and arguments that amount to untruth and avoidance. The core question is—who is 'the government' when it concerns tranquillisers?

The nub of the crime against human rights that the DoH has committed is that it has stood by throughout the years and allowed a great many thousands of people who were not sick to be turned into people who were very sick—many severely and permanently. Many of these people had not just their health taken away from them but also their relationships, their jobs, their security and their homes. Home Office figures, now no longer collected it seems, show clearly that a great many have died because of DoH inaction. The inaction continues and so does the impact on people. Withdrawal for those who are brave enough to succeed, usually without help, is not the short story that the DoH maintains that it is—it has a preface and a sequel. It may be comforting for those in the department to cherish a belief that benzodiazepines are a story of health-need met by prescription and then a return to health when the prescription ends. But the question is always does the department really believe that? Is it more a handy creed that lays no blame on manufacturers, doctors or the NHS as a whole?

All drugs carry risks is the new-age mantra of Pharma, prescribers and government, when the downside of drugs becomes apparent. This is of course a drug company formulated defence in the new world of stated medical openness. It is a way of deflecting criticism of the damage that drugs do by promoting the idea of patient responsibility—the patient should have been aware in advance. It does not seem to matter that the doctor was not aware of the possible dangers, or that Pharma emphasises only the health benefits of its products—the patient should have been imbued with a natural awareness that all drugs are dangerous and that by accepting one he was taking personal responsibility. This message carefully avoids responsibility attaching to doctors, regulators and primarily the drug companies. For Pharma it pushes away the necessity to be honest and open or to look beyond marketing strategies, for the benefit of shareholders. Manufacturers have traditionally blamed the patient first, and if that failed, then they passed the blame to doctors. And what goes around comes around. The sad element in the history of drug tragedies is that the producers of those tragedies continue to be viewed by government as honest providers of benefit to mankind, no matter how much evidence of their true behaviour emerges. But then perhaps a greater truth lies in the much repeated line from government that the pharmaceutical industry is of enormous importance to Britain.

It was not until the mid 1990s that the drug companies producing benzodiazepines, included references in their data sheets (SPCs) to show that they were highly addictive. The DoH was quite happy to accept this gross malfeasance as it is quite happy now to see the words addiction or dependence excluded from Patient Leaflets, accepting the self-serving logic of manufacturers that if these words were included, patients would be unwarrantably alarmed.

Harold Pinter, in his 2005 Nobel Laureate Acceptance Speech, asked if conscience still existed today. There is no doubt the Department of Health and those within it who are concerned with the benzodiazepine question should seriously address that point. The strategy the department has employed against critics and users of benzodiazepines over the years has been masterful. It has certainly worked and it has worked on several levels. The brilliance of the strategy has for some time centred on the offering of no active defence against individual claims of damage, but instead giving out formulaic assurances of something being done. The DoH has issued fine sounding statements and these have been designed to muddy the reality.

The policy of departmental persuasion and obfuscation is effective. Even the European Commissioner for Health seemed to have been persuaded by the official line, when campaigner Barry Haslam, through Chris Davies his MEP, took the matter to the Commission. This was the letter he received from David Byrne:

> Dear Mr and Mrs Haslam,
>
> Following our 4 February meeting on the subject of benzodiazepines, I had asked my officials to advise me on the state of play at UK and EU level. I understand that you have also subsequently spoken briefly to my officials.
>
> **The many moving letters in your dossier clearly demonstrate that the long-term use of benzodiazepines can lead to great suffering for the individuals involved. However, from the evidence available to me, it is clear that the regulatory authorities are aware of the issue of benzodiazepine dependence and their long-term adverse effects, and have been taking action on this. I understand from this review that the issue of benzodiazepine dependence and their long-term adverse effects has been under examination for at least fifteen years**.[My emphasis]
>
> In the UK, for example, the Committee on Safety of Medicines has looked at the safety of these products on a number of occasions, and issued guidance on safe prescribing in 1988. This has since been kept under review. Doctors in the UK have been reminded on various occasions about safe prescribing and the risk of dependence. Authorised product information (for healthcare professionals and patients) contains clear warnings.
>
> Indicative of the concerns which you have raised, Sir Liam Donaldson, the United Kingdom's Chief Medical Officer,

issued a Communication to Doctors regarding Patient safety and the use of Benzodiazepines following the advice of the Committee on Safety in Medicines (sic) in January 2004. This information explicitly sets out prescription advice regarding limited periods, reduced use and directs against their prescription for "mild anxiety". The issue of substance misuse is highlighted in this advice which also refers to the importance of instalment dispensing to minimise access for addicted patients.

It appears to me that this advice provides a solid basis for tackling this issue. It also suggests that the solution to this distressing problem lies in effectively implementing this advice at local level. This is clearly an issue to be pursued by the national authorities who have legal competence for the organisation and delivery of health services and which is outside the competences of the European Community.

I am grateful to you for drawing this matter to my attention. As was agreed, I enclose for your information the names of patient organisations which you may wish to contact. I am copying this letter to my colleague, Mr Erkki Liikanen who is the Commissioner with leading responsibility for pharmaceutical policy. May I once again express my appreciation for your personal dedication to the well-being of your fellow citizens—it is clearly making a real difference.

David Byrne,

Member of the European Commission, Brussels, 7 March 2004

So the Commissioner repeated back to this seasoned campaigner everything he already knew. It seemed likely that for a suitable answer, the European Commissioner had consulted the UK Department of Health for guidance. Those outside personal experience of benzodiazepines have been easily convinced that the DoH has addressed the 'problem' of tranquillisers in a serious and timely fashion: the Commissioner obviously had no idea what the problem was—non-victims seldom have.

Benzodiazepines have occasionally been referred to as a scandal, but it is the nature of that scandal and its longevity that are truly worthy of note. And the most notable aspect of both nature and longevity is the cleverly and carefully rehearsed, 'official recognition—without real recognition', that benzodiazepine addiction has received. Those with the experience of the continuing benzodiazepine 'problem' hold rather different views to those who believe benzodiazepines are a problem of the past:

> "There is a fallacy in the Western world that the benzodiazepine problem was addressed in the 1980s, particularly by the high profile campaigns, the 'That's Life' programme and other legal actions. In fact, the prescription guidelines have not been enforced for the past twenty or thirty years."
> Phil Woolas MP, Evidence to the Health Select Committee, 25 November 2004

Claims by government, that the present system of drug approval and regulation protects public health are extremely hollow when viewed against the history of tranquilliser addiction. Government ignored the epidemic in the making, until it could ignore it no longer following media revelations. Government then ignored the physical damage benzodiazepines caused, and stuck rigidly to psychiatric discussion, knowing that psychiatric labels gave high absolution from responsibility. As part of the policy of damage limitation, government underwrote the views of 'experts' such as Professor David Nutt of Bristol University, a former GSK shareholder with financial links to Wyeth and Roche who was still saying at the end of the 20th Century:

> "The case for benzodiazepine dependence causing real damage has not been made."

The risk/benefit equation with benzodiazepines is obviously extremely badly calculated but is a vital part of official camouflage. Prescribing reasons such as the ones listed below are the real reasons why many thousands have gone through the terrible physical and social agonies associated with tranquillisers. They are worth careful study:

Nursing sick wife after operation
Bereavement
Emotional upsets
After an operation
Husband's accident
Socialising
Dental pain
After-flu virus
Dry eyes
Alcohol problem
Alcoholic father
Sex abuse
Stomach trouble
Hysterectomy
Business problems
Handicapped child
Shift work
Bankruptcy
Thyroid problems
Demanding mother
Driving test
Scared of dying
Asthma
Bad fall
Rugby injury
Rape
Car crash
Headaches

Mastectomy
Interview nerves
Retirement
Dizziness
Abortion
Stroke
Shyness
Childhood insecurity
Isolation
Family problems
Floater in the eye
Broken neck
Changed job
Violent husband
Infertility
Fatal illness
Disc trouble
Divorce
Menopause
Prison
Cystitis
Cat died
Lack of confidence
Redundancy
Hay fever
Mother committed suicide
Vertigo
Jury service
Palpitations
Work pressure
Moving house
Loss of hearing
Cooker blew up
Claustrophobia
Illness
Post-natal depression
Back pain
Active/crying baby
Homelessness
Coach travel sickness

This is what the typical benzodiazepine patient leaflet has to say to patients embarking or already embarked on benzodiazepine prescriptions. Government defends this information saying it adequately protects patients:

PATIENT INFORMATION LEAFLET

DIAZEPAM TABLETS BP

Please read this leaflet carefully before you take these tablets. It briefly outlines the most important things you need to know. If you want to know more about this medicine, or you are not sure about anything, ask your doctor or your pharmacist.

The name of your medicine is Diazepam.

WHAT IS DIAZEPAM?

Diazepam tablets contain 2 mg, 5 mg or 10 mg of the active ingredient Diazepam Ph. Eur. The other ingredients are lactose, powdered cellulose, maize starch and magnesium stearate. The 5 mg tablet also contains the colours quinoline yellow (E104) and sunset yellow (El 10). The 10 mg tablet contains the colour indigo carmine (El 32).

The product is available in packs of 28 tablets

See outer packaging or the pharmacy label for contents i.e. the number of tablets.

Diazepam tablets belong to a group of drugs called benzodiazepines which promote sleep and relieve anxiety by altering brain activity concerned with emotion.

WHAT IS DIAZEPAM USED FOR?

Diazepam tablets are used for the short-term (2–4 weeks) relief of severe anxiety and tension, to relax muscles and to encourage sleep. They may also be given to relax or sedate people undergoing certain uncomfortable medical procedures. Ask your doctor or pharmacist for additional information.

BEFORE YOU TAKE DIAZEPAM

Are you sensitive to any of the ingredients in the medicine, listed above?

Have you suffered a reaction to benzodiazepines before?

Do you have long-term kidney or liver disease? Do you suffer from severe respiratory problems?

Do you suffer from Myasthenia gravis (a disorder where muscles become weak and tire easily)?

Are you taking any other sedatives e.g. temazepam, or anti-epileptic drugs e.g. phenytoin or phenobarbitone? Are you taking cimetidine or omeprazole (for stomach ulcers) or rifampicin (for tuberculosis)?

Have you had problems with alcohol or drug abuse?

Do you suffer from depression or any other psychiatric problems?

If the answer to any of these questions is YES, do not take Diazepam before consulting your doctor or pharmacist.

Do not take this medicine if you are pregnant, might become pregnant, or are breast-feeding.

If your doctor has decided that you should receive this medicine during late pregnancy or during labour, your baby might have a low body temperature, floppiness, and breathing and feeding difficulties. If this medicine is taken regularly in late pregnancy, your baby may develop withdrawal symptoms.

Your tablets may make you feel drowsy or dizzy. Do not drive or operate machinery until you are used to these tablets. You should avoid alcohol whilst taking these tablets, as it may increase the sedative effect of the drug.

TAKING DIAZEPAM

The tablets should be swallowed with a drink of water.

The usual dosage instructions are given below:

Anxiety: 2 mg three times daily. If necessary your doctor may increase the dosage.

Trouble in sleeping: 5–15 mg before bed.
Muscle spasm: Adults: 2–60 mg.
Children : 2–40 mg.

For both adults and children the dose is dependent on the symptoms, your doctor will decide on the correct dosage.

Premedication: Adults: 5–20 mg.
Children: 2–10 mg.

Your doctor will decide on the correct dosage

Elderly and Debilitated (very frail) patients:
Normally the starting dose is a half of the ordinary adult dose.

Long-term use of diazepam is not recommended. Treatment should not normally last more than 4 weeks. Your doctor has decided the dose which is suited to you. Always follow your doctor's instructions and those which are on the pharmacy label. If you do not understand these instructions, or you are in any doubt, ask your doctor or pharmacist.

You should continue to take these tablets for as long as your doctor tells you to [My emphasis]. If you forget to take a tablet, take one as soon as you remember, unless it is nearly time to take the next one. Never take two doses together. Take the remaining doses at the correct time.

If you see another doctor or go into hospital, let him or the staff know what medicines you are taking.

If you (or someone else) swallows a lot of the tablets all together, or if you think a child has swallowed any of the tablets, contact your nearest hospital casualty department or your doctor immediately.

Do not stop taking your tablets suddenly. If you do, you may suffer from withdrawal symptoms. If your doctor decides to stop your tablets, he/she will reduce the dose gradually.

When you stop taking Diazepam, you may feel anxious, depressed and restless and have difficulty sleeping. You may also experience sweating and diarrhoea. If this happens go to your doctor for advice.

AFTER TAKING DIAZEPAM

Diazepam, is taken by many patients without any problems. However, like many other medicines, it may occasionally cause side-effects in some people. These may include blurred vision, dizziness, unsteadiness and loss of co-ordination.

Rarely, confusion, feelings of excitement or depression, aggressive outbursts, skin rashes or itching, headache, stomach upset, changes in sex drive, jaundice (characterised by the yellowing of the skin or the whites of the eyes),

> difficulties in passing urine, low blood pressure and blood disorders (which may be characterised by pallor, fever or chills, sore throat, ulcers in your mouth or throat, unusual bleeding or unexplained bruising). If you have these or any other effects, whilst taking Diazepam tell your doctor immediately.
> Another side effect is daytime drowsiness. However, this effect is often mild and usually wears off after a few days treatment. If it is severe or lasts for more than a few days, tell your doctor.
> Also, if you feel unwell in any other way, tell your doctor.

It is highly doubtful that a present review of patient leaflet design will significantly alter the **almost complete fiction** set out in the current leaflets and approved by government. Note the severely limited list of possible symptoms. Note the judicious use of the word 'rarely'. How would it be possible to include realistic warnings, not hedged with 'ask your doctor', or mentioning the true reason for 2–4 weeks prescription 'normally', or listing the real dangers of side-effects? To do this would explode the carefully constructed official history of benzodiazepines and the myth of available palliative services. It is a real question as to what medical magic GPs or psychiatrists would employ to deal with such things as drug induced brain damage, other drug induced physical disabilities or indeed lost families, lost employment, homes and futures. It is the undisclosed official knowledge of the real effects associated with benzodiazepines that underlies the rigid and patently false statement—that there is help out there for patients, available in Primary and Secondary settings.

The story of benzodiazepine addiction then, is one of drug company power and influence in government and the healthcare system. It is one of a regulatory system that did not work even after the Thalidomide tragedy and of government dependence on that failing system.

When the real impact on real people of benzodiazepines was forced onto government and the regulatory agencies by patients and the media, the story became one of political calculation about possible fallout. The considerations included political cost, economic realities, the image of the NHS, the lack of alternatives to benzodiazepines and the unique position of doctors as independent contractors.

In order to marginalise the scandal and avoid responsibility for the damage, a policy of seeming action and public reassurance was instituted. A list of approved responses was drawn up to respond to critics, patients and the media. It did not matter what information was laid before government departments, the response was kept to the same pre-formulated message and if this avoided any reference to points being made, it did not matter. To engage in debate about the realities being described was seen as a possible opening of the floodgates to discovery. The drug company line of blaming the patient where possible was followed. It did not matter that benzodiazepines had been prescribed mainly for personal problems not illnesses—the line of departments and agencies was that all prescriptions had been properly aimed at anxiety. This was seen as a great strength in future strategies. A psychiatric label is permanent and draws unique conclusions in the public mind.

If at any time it was impossible to maintain the line that a prescription had been properly issued for anxiety, patients were referred to their doctor's responsibility. Stories in the media giving the impression that there were a few (rather than a large number) of ignorant doctors damaging health and ignoring official advice, were seen as fortunately missing the point.

The Department of Health, its regulatory agencies and government generally, slowly began to cover the tracks by issuing guidance to doctors and later to local health bodies on appropriate prescribing. The setting up of PCTs, SHAs, NICE and the guidance given to doctors by the CSM, and others later meant that direct responsibility was now avoidable—all criticism and claims could now be redirected to doctors and local health authorities. But in addition it also meant that the entire impression could be given to the media and others, that government had acted responsibly. It also enabled Health Minister Rosie Winterton at the DoH in 2004, to continue to tell campaigners that the priority of government was to prevent addiction occurring in the first place. Medically-induced benzodiazepine addiction has now become old news and the present government has been able to successfully persuade itself that it has fulfilled any responsibilities it might have. Ironically government probably does not understand that to benzodiazepine veterans, the strategies and statements at present being employed with SSRIs are following an old score.

There has been no government ownership of responsibility so has the patient any representation in a failing system? Just as the statements on benzodiazepines from health sources are ultimately empty of meaning, so too are statements from politicians who achieve a position in government from where they could have altered the situation. These are the two letters to Barry Haslam, one from David Blunkett MP and the other from Paul Boateng MP on the subject of tranquillisers, written as you will note some time ago. Needless to say the 'national scandal' has never been addressed. Neither has 'justice' been obtained. These politicians while out of power, expressed concern, but in power did nothing.

> Dear Mr Haslam,
> Thank you for your recent letter regarding Benzodiazepine Tranquillisers.

> Dawn Primarolo and myself have been taking up cases and have advised on how best the groups involved might organise a parliamentary lobby and keep attention on these issues.
> We have also tried to assist through both Parliamentary Questions and raising the matter on the floor of the House, in pushing the Government to accept its own responsibilities and to take action now to ensure that it does not happen again.
> This is something we will be returning to both in the House and in terms of our own future policy development.
> I am passing your letter to Paul Boateng who, as the legal affairs spokesman, has specific responsibility for the litigation side of what is a national scandal.
> David Blunkett MP, Shadow Secretary of State for Health,
> 24 February 1994

> Dear Mr Haslam
> Your letter to David Blunkett has been passed to me. The case of the Ativan victims is one on which I have been very active in recent months. I am therefore, of course, always glad to receive any research papers to supplement the large number of such documents that I have in my possession. I thank you for those which you have sent to me thus far and would be grateful for anything further. Clearly, the aim of all involved in this sorry affair is the provision of justice to the victims of these drugs.
> Paul Boateng MP, 25 April 1994

'Normal,' for thousands of the iatrogenic-dependent, ingesting these prescribed tablets in good faith, is in reality a gross reduction in the quality of their life. With mental, physical and emotional capabilities restricted, these patients find their world contracts, as they become unable to solve problems in life, unable to empathise with family and friends, unable to be interested in the world outside, developing obsessions, developing agoraphobia, prone to irrational outbursts of rage, beset by inexplicable physical symptoms.

It takes a person who had a strong mind before starting on tranquillisers to withdraw successfully (and from the subsequent antidepressants frequently prescribed in an attempt to minimise the depression triggered by the benzodiazepines). It needs the ability to take advantage of any moments of clarity in which to contemplate a life without a customary bedside or pocket bottle of tablets. Through no fault of their own, that bottle of tablets became their life support system.

For many it takes a high degree of willpower to face the symptoms of withdrawal. Rebound insomnia, the intense muscle and joint pain, the baffling sensory sensations affecting nerves all over the body, sleep apnoea, tinnitus, the irrational outbursts of rage, the nausea, the mood swings, are just a few of the horrendous and well-documented series of benzodiazepine withdrawal symptoms.

It takes a very strong family or strong support network to endure this journey through the unknown with the iatrogenic addict. If the whole process is successful and a drugs free personality reappears, they and the recovered addict have to learn to relate to each other again. Repairing relationships can take many years, if it is possible at all. Withdrawing from the drug can take years and there is the possibility of failure.

Hundreds of millions of taxpayers' money is spent to benefit users of illegal drugs, increasingly including benzodiazepines. The almost empty list of government activities in regard to legal addicts is pitiful, after forty-seven years of damage inflicted on the trusting. If alterations to regulations could be considered to allow instalment prescribing, why could they not be considered to control doctors' prescribing? If the daily creation of new iatrogenic addicts by uninformed doctors was actively prevented, the pleas for money to be put into support networks would gradually cease.

It would seem then that for the Department of Health, benzodiazepine addiction is little understood (or perhaps deliberately misunderstood) and any understanding is actively avoided. **Convincing policy-makers that it is not the patients who misuse the drugs, but the drugs which misuse the patients has thus far proved to be an impossible task.**

Is there a defence for the incalculable health damage inflicted on UK citizens through benzodiazepines? Professor Heather Ashton does not believe so, and neither do patients. 'Power and Dependence', gives a clear analysis of the history of benzodiazepines up to the late 1980s. The book description included the following:

> "...the risks [of benzodiazepines] were always obvious and...the providers of medicine between them, readily let this happen."

Government, civil servants and regulators, maintaining silence, eschewing debate and making no attempt to verify patient claims, have been avoiding all aspects of responsibility for what they allowed to happen since the first claims of harm emerged following licensing of the drugs. The gloss that has been placed on what must surely be the greatest single source of medical damage ever inflicted by a healthcare system has been accepted by most. But then how many of them studied the daily life of a withdrawing benzodiazepine addict? Most people will never have intimately known an addict before he became one. Most of us will never have to ask ourselves this question, “How would I feel if everything I had hoped for and could have become was taken away needlessly?” How much worse would it be, knowing that you had done nothing personally to make that happen beyond holding a misplaced belief in the expertise of medicine?

Benzodiazepine damage has been and is still a great evil in the world. How should we view the producers of the scandal and the unaccountable who have maintained it? Benzodiazepine campaigners and patients face Westminster politicians whose main concerns are the risk of losing their cars and red boxes, or the possibility of acquiring such things. What does individual justice mean in the minds of men and women with such thoughts?

The Influence of the Pharmaceutical Industry
House of Commons Health Committee 2004–05

In 2004–2005 The House of Commons Health Select Committee conducted an inquiry into the Influence of the Pharmaceutical Industry. The following is a summary of their findings on the UK Drugs Regulator:

> "The interests of pharmaceutical companies and those of the public, patients and the NHS often overlap but they are not identical...
>
> An effective regulatory regime to ensure that the industry works in the public interest is essential. Unfortunately, the present regulatory system is failing to provide this...
>
> Over-prescription of the COX-2 inhibitors, Vioxx and Celebrex, has been linked to thousands of deaths and many more cases of heart failure. These cases illustrate a series of failures. Manufacturers are known to have suppressed certain trials for these drugs in the US and may have done the same in the UK. In addition, there were inadequacies in the licensing and post-marketing surveillance procedures and excessive promotion of the drugs to doctors...
>
> The industry is by no means solely to blame for the difficulties we describe. The regulators and prescribers are also open to criticism. The regulator, the Medicines and Healthcare products Regulatory Agency (MHRA), has failed to adequately scrutinise licensing data and its post-marketing surveillance is inadequate. The MHRA Chairman stated that trust is integral to effective regulation, but trust, while convenient, may mean that the regulatory process is not strict enough. The organisation has been too close to the industry, a closeness underpinned by common policy objectives, agreed processes, frequent contact, consultation and interchange of staff...

> In view of the failings of the MHRA, we recommend a fundamental review of the organisation in order to ensure that safe and effective medicines, with necessary prescribing constraints are licensed. "

Core recommendations were as follows:

362. Our inquiry revealed major failing in the regulatory system. The organisation, process and techniques of the MHRA are focussed on bringing drugs to market fast. The stated rationale—that patients benefit from new drugs—is insufficiently qualified by consideration of relative merit or value or therapeutic need.

363. The process by which drugs are licensed is far from transparent. There is no public access to the data presented by the pharmaceutical companies, or to the assessments undertaken by the MHRA. There is not enough involvement of patients, the public and the wider scientific community, and the Agency does not listen or communicate well. After years of intense secrecy surrounding UK drug regulation, we welcome the MHRA's commitment to improve external communications, and to give patients a greater voice, but we are not convinced that these changes will be sufficient to counter the current inadequate state of affairs. We recommend that the MHRA publishes, in some form of useable database, the material it receives from drug companies and the assessments it sends to advisory bodies at the time it sends them.

364. The MHRA does not routinely examine raw data submitted with the licence application but is dependent on summaries provided by the applicant. The Expert Working Group on SSRIs report of December 2004 showed that summaries of information may not provide the detail required to assess drug risks adequately. The licensing process relies excessively on the results of trials designed and presented by companies, in the absence of independent input. Trial design and the way in which results are evaluated and reported can obscure negative results. More checks and balances on the part of the regulator would serve to reassure the public of the stringency of the licensing procedure. The MHRA should put in place systematic procedures to randomly audit raw data. The results of such audits should be published...Guidance should be provided by the MHRA to the industry as to the types of clinical trial likely to prove the degree of therapeutic gain...

366. **The adverse drug reactions reported in the clinical trials that are considered in the medicines licensing process typically prove unreliable as a guide to routine clinical practice. Moreover, the**

adverse effects that may be linked to stopping treatment are insufficiently investigated. [My emphasis] The MHRA should focus more intensely on updating drug benefit/risk profiles in the Summary of Product Characteristics, following systematic post-marketing review.

368. Drug manufacturers provide less funding for Phase IV trials than for pre-marketing trials, possibly because such avenues of research are not profitable. The types of thorough, comparative studies needed to determine long-term efficacy, tolerance and risk of side-effects in large populations are therefore not undertaken. Independent research into these areas is limited.

369. **Overwhelming evidence is required by the regulator before drug warnings are proposed** [My emphasis] or when drugs may be withdrawn, Only 19 drugs have been withdrawn between 1993 and 2004. On the other hand, medicines can be licensed in the absence of adequate data or investigation into possible adverse reactions and with proof of only limited therapeutic value. We agree that it is in the public interest to allow access to potentially life-saving therapy as quickly as possible, but **timely withdrawal or provision of strict guidance on medicines that are dangerous if inappropriately prescribed is an equally life-saving pursuit**. [My emphasis] We recommend that the MHRA is given the same authority to propose restrictions on drug use as it has when approving drugs.

370. The recent review of the Yellow Card Scheme has led to a welcome increase in public access to information gleaned from the system and to the introduction of pilot schemes of patient reporting of suspected adverse reactions. However, we are concerned that these measures will not address the main failings of the Yellow Card Scheme. The rate of adverse drug effects reported by healthcare professionals is inadequate, and when they are reported they are not always investigated or pursued with sufficient robustness. We recommend that:

- the system of patient reporting to the Yellow Card Scheme be put in place countrywide as soon as possible;
- steps be taken to improve rates of healthcare professional reporting of adverse drug reactions;
- greater efforts be made to investigate signals of possible problems; and
- that maximum transparency be combined with concerted efforts to explain the uncertainties of risk

371. After a drug is withdrawn for health reasons, there are often a number of questions in the public mind, not least because such cases typically leave behind victims injured by the drug or bereaved relatives of people who suffered fatal reactions to the drug, as well as people who are denied access to a drug they may have found beneficial. A public inquiry could answer such questions as: should the safety problems have been better predicted from the pre-market testing data? Did the regulators get full and appropriate safety and efficacy data from the manufacturer? Was the right judgement made in balancing the risks and benefits of the drug? Could the health problem with the drug have been identified and acted upon earlier? Could and should the drug have been withdrawn earlier? Was sufficient consideration given to the continued provision of the drug for patients who uniquely benefited from it after withdrawal? Such a public inquiry could not only provide understanding and a sense of justice for the public, but equally importantly would ensure that the drug regulatory agency can learn effectively from mistakes and avoid them in the future. We recommend that there should be a public inquiry whenever a drug is withdrawn on health grounds.

375. The MHRA, like many regulatory organisations, is entirely funded by fees from those it regulates. However, unlike many regulators, it competes with other European agencies for fee income. This situation has led to concerns that it may lose sight of the need to protect and promote public health above all else as it seeks to win fee income from the companies. No evidence was submitted with proposals for a better system for funding the MHRA, but it is important to be aware of the dangers of the present arrangements. These dangers make our other recommendations for improving the regulatory system all the more important.

The government response to the committee's findings on the regulatory system came in September 2005. Two of the responses are worth noting to gain a picture of the seriousness of government concern about patient safety. First the government recognises no real problems with the MHRA:

> "The Government appreciates that it may appear that the roles of promoting health and representing the interests of the pharmaceutical industry in the same department may not serve the public as well as it should. However, the interests of patients and the industry are not exclusive. Having a strong industry that is properly regulated by the MHRA brings benefits to patients, the NHS, and the wider community. Patients benefit by receiving innovative medicines, which have

saved the lives of thousands of patients who may have died in the past from diseases such as cancer or coronary heart disease. The NHS benefits through its clinicians being recognised as world leaders in research, and through the resources it receives for carrying out clinical trials. It is this positive environment that makes the pharmaceutical industry invest in the UK, and it is important that these roles be brought together in a balanced and effective way. The Government believes that at present the Department of Health is the right place to balance all of these interests..."

"The MHRA has a dedicated team of multidisciplinary staff in place which focuses on newly licensed products...
The Government does not support the recommendation that consideration should be given to the establishment of post-marketing surveillance and drug safety monitoring systems independently of the Licensing Authority as this would impede the continuous examination of the risk/benefit balance...[My emphasis**]**

You would be forgiven for wondering if the department had read anything the Health Committee wrote, or read any of the evidence it had heard and received. The response addressed no concerns and recognised no problems with the existing system of regulation, which had clearly been shown to be a failing one. The disregard for the evidence is succinctly contained in the second sentence:

"Having a strong industry that is properly regulated by the MHRA brings benefits to patients, the NHS, and the wider community."

No one would argue with that except for the fact that the Health Committee had demonstrated two things beyond doubt:

- The industry was already too strong and had too much influence on UK health policy, and
- The MHRA had singularly failed to regulate that industry

What value to place on the government argument that the one depended on the other? In reply to criticisms regarding the amount of independent information available to doctors, the government said:

"The Government agrees that clinicians should receive independent advice on medicines. Guidance and advice is

> offered at national and local level already from local Drugs and Therapeutics Committees and from NICE respectively. In addition, the Department of Health purchases the Drug and Therapeutics Bulletin (DTB) for all NHS doctors in England. The DTB is an independent eight-page bulletin, published monthly by the Consumers' Association. It provides critical impartial reviews of treatments."

Less than nine months after making this assurance regarding the DTB, the government suddenly announced that it would no longer fund it. The Parliamentary record Hansard from 12 June 2006, reports on the reply to a question in the House of Lords as to why this was. Health Minister, Lord Warner maintained:

> "The decision not to renew the Department of Health's national contract for distribution of the Drug and Therapeutics Bulletin was informed by our policy to devolve as much responsibility as possible to the National Health Service and to look very critically at central spending. It is our policy that central spending should be kept to an absolute minimum to maximise the resources available for the NHS to manage at local level. The decision also took account of the availability of other sources of medicines information. They include the British National Formulary; National Prescribing Centre information and advice, which include coverage of new medicines; National Institute for Health and Clinical Excellence clinical guidance; the wealth of information available through the National Library for Health; and various academic and professional journals..."

Was this really a policy to devolve responsibility or a reaction to criticisms made by the editor of the DTB at the Health Committee? A reduction in the amount of independent information available to doctors seems to be what the government wished to achieve, after asserting in response to the committee that such information was vital. It demonstrates once again, political indifference to important ways of protecting patients and perhaps a more murky influence.

The Dark World of Medical Unaccountability

"Morality? What has morality to do with the law?
Sir Abraham Haphazard, The Barchester Chronicles,
(BBC 1982)

"If this case [Vioxx] can't get into the courts here, then I don't know what will. There's a real chance that we will simply end up in some mid-Atlantic limbo land where we can't get funding here, we can't get the cases going here and at the same time we get thrown out in the US. So British people end up with no justice, no recompense, whereas in the States there's a very strong feeling that Merck will settle these cases."
Martyn Day, Leigh Day & Co Solicitors, London 2005

Manslaughter by gross negligence

"Negligence is generally defined as failure to exercise a reasonable level of precaution given the circumstances and so may include both acts and omissions. The defendants in such cases are often people carrying out jobs that require special skills or care, such as doctors who fail to meet the standard which could be expected from them and cause death. In R v Bateman (1925) 19 Cr App.R. 8, the Court of Criminal Appeal held that gross negligence manslaughter involved the following elements:

1. the defendant owed a duty to the deceased to take care
2. the defendant breached this duty
3. the breach caused the death of the deceased
4. the defendant's negligence was gross, that is, it showed such a disregard for the life and safety of others as to amount to a crime and deserve punishment."

Negligence

"Failure to exercise the care toward others which would reasonably be expected of a person in the circumstances, or

taking action which a reasonable person would not. Failure to exercise care, resulting in injury to others."
Legal Definitions on the Internet

On 22 June 2007, a newspaper article greeted the reader with the headline that more than one in five junior doctors was suicidal because of a government recruitment fiasco. Some ninety-four per cent reported higher stress levels than normal. A third said they had drunk more in the past six months and others were experiencing symptoms of anxiety, depression, sleep disturbance, a sense of hopelessness, less fulfilling sex, lack of appetite and tearfulness. Stories such as this make the news. The 17,000 (perhaps many more) whose deaths have been linked to benzodiazepines and the uncounted thousands of people whose lives have been destroyed through ill health caused by benzodiazepines do not make headlines.

Many of the prescription drugs licensed in this country are exactly the same drugs as those licensed in the US. Most of what is known about the machinations of the manufacturers of those drugs comes from the US and much of it is disclosed through legal actions in that country. The UK does not do legal actions against drug companies—Vioxx is the latest case in point. But that situation came about because of a failed legal action against the manufacturers of benzodiazepines in the late 1980s—principally Wyeth and Roche.

At the end of the 1980s a group action began over tranquilliser damage involving thousands of claimants, which eventually cost the Legal Aid Board around £45 million. The principal claim was that the companies were aware of the dangers of addiction and other side-effects before making this information available to prescribers and patients. Roche and Wyeth denied this, and the action was discontinued in 1994 after the Board withdrew the funding for those involved in the action. This was because there were a large number of cases where there were serious difficulties with causation. It was also on the basis that substantial costs had been incurred and a large number of cases were likely to generate only a modest level of damages. It was therefore, in the opinion of the Board, not worthwhile for the legal aid to continue. It is worth noting that the formula it used for working out likely damages was completely flawed, both as regards the inadequate period of time recognized for health damage and the nature of that damage. This myth surrounding benzodiazepine damage was the creation of Pharma and the Department of Health.

The resources of the defendant drug companies Roche and Wyeth had made certain that the cases dragged on. The Conservative government of the time made the decision that this should never happen again. Saving public money was given precedence over ensuring that the law could defend UK patients against the rapacious activities of drug manufacturers, whose products the UK government licensed. They did two things:

1. They set up the Legal Services Commission to replace the Legal Aid Board. The LSC acts as a quasi court. After determining income levels, the LSC calculates the amount of likely damages before determining whether the amount of legal aid would exceed that figure. Since the law is based on the now dismissed reality of a few months of withdrawal and problem over, the legal aid figure required always exceeds the damages figure. Therefore there is no legal aid.
2. To offset (they said) a likely reduction in access to justice, the government introduced the No-win, No-fee system. But this did not lead to access to compensation for tranquilliser addicts for the simple reason that such cases would prove intractable and costly given the resources of drug companies.

At the end of 2005, Martyn Day, a solicitor involved with Vioxx claimants confirmed that legal aid for group actions against drug companies had been massively cut back in recent years. The No-win, No-fee arrangements—known as conditional fee agreements—had been ostensibly meant to take up the slack. But insurance against losing and having to pay the drug company's costs is hard to get and prohibitively expensive. In the Vioxx case, the costs of losing were estimated at £5m.

Lord Brennan QC, a Deputy High Court judge expressed the opinion that people injured by prescribed drugs would no longer be able to mount claims for compensation in UK courts. The five hundred people who had had strokes or heart attacks following treatment with the withdrawn painkiller Vioxx had lost their appeal against the LSC refusal to grant legal aid. Almost 500,000 people in the UK were taking Vioxx when its US producers Merck removed it from sale in 2004. The case against Merck was a strong one and quite possibly might have been potentially much more successful than the benzodiazepine group action.

Although Merck had tried to make it seem as though its withdrawal of Vioxx was motivated by concern for public health, the evidence does not point in that direction. Analysts believe the decision had more to do with the health of Merck's finances and the fact that the lawsuits in the US were building up. The evidence showed that Merck actually wanted to broaden the market for COX-2 inhibitors. This was a re-run of GSK's attempt to broaden the use of Seroxat as an antidepressant for children. As in that case, Merck's attempt backfired.

In November 2004, FDA Safety Officer Dr David Graham appeared before the US Senate Finance Committee. In Dr. Graham's opinion, even using Merck's own trials data, some 88,000 to 139,000 had suffered heart attacks as a result of taking Vioxx in America alone and of that number,

30% to 40% had probably died. He likened the situation to 500 to 900 aircraft dropping from the sky:

> "This translates to two to four aircraft every week, week in and week out, for the past 5 years. If you were confronted by this situation, what would be your reaction?"

In a press release Merck had stated that the drug was being withdrawn despite its belief that:

> "It would have been possible to continue to market Vioxx with labelling that would incorporate these new data..."

The APPROVe trial which Merck carried out may have had less to do with safety and more to do with gaining FDA approval for using Vioxx as a prevention treatment against colon polyps. Had the three year study not been halted by the Data Safety Monitoring Board for safety reasons, Vioxx might well still be on the market and the heart attack toll still rising.

On February 13 1992, the consumer charity Social Audit said that more than 10,000 hospital beds are constantly occupied by people suffering from the side-effects of prescribed drugs. The claim was based on four studies between 1981 and 1988 suggesting that adverse reactions to drugs were to blame for between three and five per cent of admissions. The cost to the National Health Service of the side-effects of cardiovascular, arthritis and ulcer medicines and antibiotics was up to £1 billion a year. Charles Medawar described how the receivers of drugs were kept in ignorance of risks associated with them, doctors were influenced by drug salesmen and the Committee on Safety of Medicines worked in secret and was staffed by people who had financial links to drug companies. As an example of official complacency, he pointed to the statement made in 1980 by the drugs watchdog of the time, the Committee on the Review of Medicines. The statement said that nationally there were only twenty-eight cases of dependence associated with benzodiazepines between 1960 and 1977. As Medawar said:

> "Anyone taking the drugs would have known that was balderdash."

The legal reality for the many thousands of patients who suffered hypnotic and tranquilliser damage due to over-prescription and the activities of the manufacturers goes something like this:

Many were first prescribed these drugs in the 1960s and 70s and many were, in ignorance, prescribed other drugs, to deal with symptoms produced by the benzodiazepines. This fact of course was a boon to the manufacturers, and as the law stands, it is very difficult to prove cause and effect, when a variety of drugs are involved. The law does not recognize common themes—ten thousand people can take a drug and report similar experiences as a result, but that has no currency in UK law, particularly with drugs marketed as psychotropic medication.

Those who became aware of what the drugs were doing to their lives often withdrew without medical encouragement or help, a process which can extend over several years. Benzodiazepines frequently produce severe and debilitating physical and psychiatric symptoms while they are being taken. They are not only drugs which are notoriously hard to withdraw from but they also produce a new range of symptoms during the withdrawal process. Many people never recover their health, and many find they have been cast adrift in society, without jobs and security. There are those who lost their jobs through the effects of the drugs while they were taking them, but ironically there are also those who first became unable to work because of the severity of the withdrawal symptoms. Some people have been unable to work for decades with an obvious impact on family life and economic well-being. But the government does not recognize this situation and the law provides no redress for this state-induced situation.

Since the group action against the manufacturers, various guidelines were issued by them as to prescription. For example, it was recommended in the late 1980s by Roche, the manufacturer of Valium that it should only be prescribed for a maximum of 4 weeks. Having issued these guidelines, the manufacturers were able to produce benzodiazepines with legal impunity, effectively passing the responsibility wholly to those who did the prescribing. There, patients hit another snag—legal aid to sue a doctor was now unlikely to be forthcoming because of false assessments of damage caused and therefore inadequate figures of damages likely to be awarded. Finding a solicitor to take a case on a contingency basis was extremely difficult and the wholly unknown number who have managed to extract some degree of damages, have not done so in court, but have been given them by doctors' insurance companies based on a perceived threat of success.

A handy legal fiction has been maintained that before the second part of the 1980s, GPs and psychiatrists were quite justified in not being aware of the extent of the addictiveness of benzodiazepines, in spite of a mountain of independent research from around the world and patient reporting that clearly demonstrated how addictive they were. Professor Heather Ashton, Charles Medawar and others have condemned the gullibility of drug regulators and doctors for thinking benzodiazepines were non-addictive tranquillisers. As Medawar has said:

> "First it was alcohol and opium; then morphine, cocaine and heroin; then chloral, bromides and barbiturates—until it was the turn of the benzodiazepines."

Now it is the turn of SSRIs.

But the Committee on the Safety of Medicines did not issue guidelines to doctors until 1988 and so Pharma, having taken itself out of the frame by making sure the group action failed, and having subsequently issued prescription advice, was now followed by doctors who were absolved from any responsibility for their prescribing practices before 1988.

Anyone who had been taking the drugs for ten, twenty years or more, before 1988, saw all responsibility dissolve. Many who had no idea what was going on and only withdrew much later, found themselves being told that all the damage done to their health would have been done by the time the CSM guidelines were issued. Significantly no legal weight is attached to economic impact—extra years after 1988 for those who were not able to work, apparently do not count as further damage.

It might be imagined that those patients who were over-prescribed post 1988, would find it easier to take legal action against a doctor for his actions, but the difficulties with legal aid still apply, including the degree of recognized damage. Doctors by and large still escape from and avoid their theoretical responsibilities implied in the concept of 'duty of care'.

Breach of Duty

There are now clear guidelines as to addictiveness of benzodiazepine drugs. A GP should be under a duty to offer a withdrawal programme, to very gradually reduce the daily dosage with very regular GP reviews at the surgery. As an alternative, he could refer the dependent patient to an appropriate withdrawal support network or a psychiatric department, to manage a withdrawal programme.

In fact there are no dedicated withdrawal facilities in existence today, few voluntary organisations, and psychiatrists are not keen to take on iatrogenic addicts. In addition, most GPs remain ignorant about withdrawal protocols and have little inclination or time to offer regular encouragement and advice to the addicts they created. If GPs after 1988 failed to attempt those steps that theoretically constituted a reasonable standard of care there have been few consequences. The reality is that many GPs not only ignore the guidelines on prescribing, but do not offer what would be reasonably seen as 'duty of care'. Yet it is still inordinately difficult for knowledgeable patients to secure redress. Why is this so?

Anyone applying for public funding for a clinical negligence claim must now go through the NHS complaints procedure first. It seems more than reasonable to suspect that government and the NHS wish people to become so embroiled within the complaints process, without access to independent support and advice that they fall away—never emerging to become a drain on the public purse, however deserving their claim.

Causation

Those patients who were prescribed before 1988 might think that after 1988, continuing prescriptions and hence continuing harm would constitute negligence, but this does not follow. It has to be shown that any GP negligence caused further harm beyond that which had already taken place by 1988. Clearly this is a virtual impossibility. The legal view is that by 1988 a benzodiazepine may have been prescribed for several years so at that point it would be highly likely that the full potential of withdrawal symptoms would have been reached by that date. The same potential for residual symptoms would also have already have been acquired. This is a view which has no scientific basis and it would be more than interesting to know where it came from.

There is one final legal hurdle the patient has to overcome. For potential claims the usual rule is that he must issue proceedings within 3 years of a negligent act or the date of his knowledge of that negligent act. But usually patients find that their pleas of justified ignorance due to lack of information are not taken into account and are not believed, nor is the fact that benzodiazepines often take away the ability to think, and can take years to recover from.

So the situation was that government agencies licensed the drugs, based on trial summaries from the drug companies. The membership of the licensing body had their careers linked to manufacturers and these regulators did not insist that companies carried out post-marketing safety studies, even when patients were making it obvious that there were serious safety concerns.

In 1988 when the Regulator finally got around to issuing guidelines, there was no insistence that doctors review the vast numbers of dependent patients they already had, so they were never given the choice of withdrawal. The Regulator (it subsequently claimed) had no power or responsibility to enforce or monitor the effectiveness of guidelines. Patient Leaflets remained anodyne, giving patients no information about common and serious side-effects.

What course was left when those patients who managed to discover what had happened to them and why, justifiably sought redress for their grievances? The answer should have been the law, but the judicial process is virtually impossible to access. It was certainly game, set and match to the drug manufacturers, the medical establishment, prescribers, and the politicians who knew that the licensing system was seriously flawed, that doctors were not controlled, and huge numbers of patients were affected.

Pharmaceutical companies, government politicians and medicine have a unique immunity from legal and ethical responsibility in the UK. Big Pharma has consistently demonstrated that avarice is its guiding star and not the welfare of the people that democratic government theoretically protects. The money it makes provides it with armour against all consequences. There is no will in the corridors of power to initiate change. Instead, by dogged obfuscation and deliberate misunderstanding, government supports the bringers of harm, making them inviolate.

Patient safety is dependent upon a system of licensing and regulation which consistently fails to curb the excesses of drug marketing and which recognizes no responsibility for the policing and use of drugs it gives doctors the ability to prescribe. Patients bear the consequences, remain largely uninformed and are unaware of the background to widespread medical injury. There is no redress.

There is a myth in the uneducated public mind that government cares for individuals, their freedom and their safety—that a scandal will be recognized and addressed, even if belatedly. But government does not care to enforce an efficient working system of protection in the provision of medicines. Government does not believe that patients should have easier access to the law. Government believes in individual protection only when that function coincides with its own agenda and does not conflict with it.

Pharma Goes To Market

"The pharmaceutical industry is immensely powerful. It is one of the most profitable of industries, truly global, and closely connected to politicians, particularly in the United States. Compared with it, medicine is a disorganised mess. Doctors have become dependent on the industry in a way that undermines their independence and ability to do their best by patients."
British Medical Journal, 2005

"There is indeed an extraordinary entanglement between drug companies and the medical profession. On the one hand the drug industry develops new drugs and promotes drug use in order to make money. On the other hand the medical profession prescribes these drugs in order to help people. One might think that there would be a healthy symbiotic relationship between these two organisations. But sadly there is emerging evidence that this is not the case and that the relationship is especially unhealthy in the case of drugs used for mental ill health. This situation stems from faults on both sides, and also from government policy."
Professor C. Heather Ashton, DM, FRCP
'The Role of the Pharmaceutical Companies in the Treatment of Mental Ill Health', May 18 2007

Pharmaceutical companies are seemingly Teflon organisations—no revelation of their egregious activities sticks, which is not surprising given their proven ability to manipulate and control law, regulators, governments and the media. The personality diagnostic checklist in DSM IV and the World Health Organisation ICD 10 lead to the inescapable conclusion—reached by Dr Robert Hare, FBI consultant on psychopaths, that if corporations were individuals, they would demonstrate all the characteristics of the psychopath. And Drug Companies are of course among the most profitable corporations on the planet. Hare says these are the psychopathic characteristics demonstrated by the Corporation:

1. Callous unconcern for the feelings of others.
2. Incapacity to maintain enduring relationships.

3. Reckless disregard for the safety of others.
4. Deceitfulness, repeated lying and conning others for profit.
5. Inability to experience guilt.
6. Failure to conform to social norms with respect to lawful behaviour.

Four of the world's biggest pharmaceutical companies, Johnson & Johnson, Pfizer, Novartis and Procter & Gamble are in 2007, feverishly lobbying in Europe for authority to launch a new digital Pharmaceutical television channel, ostensibly as a way to give patients more information—empowering them in modern phraseology. Achievement of this goal would necessitate the European authorities abandoning the long-standing restrictions aimed at protecting patients and would require changes to the regulations that ban all direct-to-consumer advertising of medicinal drugs. The proposed interactive channel would be funded by the industry, just as the UK drug regulator the MHRA is, and would carry detailed information from drug companies about their products.

The industry has been lobbying the European Commission for some years to be allowed direct access to patients. It trots out the usual argument that lifting restrictions would improve competitiveness and innovation and at the same time makes the usual threatening announcement (usually wheeled out at the slightest sign of a desire to control its practices), that companies may relocate to the US where things are done differently.

The International Society of Drug Bulletins (ISDB) says that in both the US and New Zealand, where companies are allowed to advertise directly to patients, the practice has led to poorer health for patients but to much greater profits for Pharma.

> "The drug industry's onslaught of advertising to promote prescription drugs...does not promote public health and increases costs and unnecessary prescriptions, more than 200 US medical school professors said last week. In the United States the industry spends $4bn (£2.3bn; €3.3bn) a year on direct to consumer advertising."
> Jeanne Lenzer, British Medical Journal, 5 November 2005

The reaction of drug companies and their trade unions to sincere and accurate observations like this is of course to deny the truth. They produce one of their other stock arguments, used for a variety of situations, which is that direct to consumer advertising is educational at a time when there is significant under-diagnosis and under-treatment of diseases that affect millions of people. Under-diagnosed conditions include the neglected millions who are depressed, suffer from ADHD, Restless Legs Syndrome, Sexual Dysfunction and so on.

> "Pharmaceutical companies' messages are focused on relatively few top sellers, exaggerating effects and concealing risks, confusing patients and putting pressure on doctors to prescribe drugs they would not use otherwise."
> The International Society of Drug Bulletins

Professor C.H. Ashton recalls that a pharmacologist working for Sanofi Pharmaceuticals once said:

> "In the beginning, the pharmaceutical industry was run by chemists...This was not so bad. [But] now most of them are run by people with MBAs, or things like that, people who could be the chief executive of Renault, Volvo or anything. They don't know about drugs."

The marketeers may not know anything about chemistry but they certainly understand influence, control and where the market is. If the indication for a discovered chemical compound is not there, it must be created—in other words a disease suitable for the drug must be invented. Big Pharma is exceedingly good at doing that.

In the 1970s Upjohn came across a variation of the existing benzodiazepine creation, and produced Xanax. It was then faced with the problem of how to maximise its sales potential. There was a great deal of confusion at this time as to the definition of anxiety. Upjohn and the psychiatrists in the American Psychiatric Association working on the Diagnostic and Statistical Manual (DSM III) came up with a new and separate anxiety category—panic disorder for which Xanax amazingly was ideally suited. The isolation of panic disorder as a separate entity may have had something to do with the fact that 60–100% of the panel members had financial ties to various drug companies.

Anxiety is still split into separate categories which include panic disorder, agoraphobia, social phobia and generalised anxiety disorder. But anyone who is familiar with the field should know that all these categories overlap. The new compartmentalisation produced by the pharma-linked psychiatrists was handy in that it allowed a new marketing opportunity for drug companies, who used it to push the message that their me-too drug targeted specific anxiety disorders. In fact all the benzodiazepine drugs act as tranquillisers, sedate in the same way and all work on the various manifestations of anxiety. The marketing of Xanax was deliberately designed to take advantage of the medical profession's pharma-promoted confusion surrounding the classification of anxiety disorders.

The manufacturers of benzodiazepines sold the drugs to doctors and regulators as virtually side-effect free. The great majority of doctors and the regulators saw only that the drugs were less dangerous in overdose than the barbiturates and looked no further. Neither regulators nor most doctors ever stopped to consider the complete lack of evidence on long-term side-effects. Neither did they ever seem to consider the possibility that dependence/addiction might figure among these. Those who claimed scientific expertise should have considered the potential for addiction but instead they ignored it and most prescribing doctors easily succumbed to the glossy benzodiazepine adverts in medical journals and to the educational message coming from drug representatives. For a time benzodiazepines became the most commonly prescribed drugs in the world.

It was patients not doctors who discovered the addiction, but the drug companies fought a long and protracted rearguard action, being helped by the lack of effective regulatory action, their access to doctors and the indifference of the Department of Health. It is now nearly thirty years since doctors were warned about the lack of evidence on long-term efficacy and nearly twenty since they were told that the only safe prescribing was short-term. But today the legacy of Pharma influence is still to be found in the huge number of medically dependent patients in the UK.

The tranquilliser star waned as all medical drug-ascendency does. Pharma can always be relied upon to move the goal posts and blitz prescribers and regulators with something ostensibly new and improved as a replacement. As benzodiazepine prescriptions fell, along came the Z drugs—zopiclone, zolpidem, zaleplon and eszopiclone (Lunesta). These drugs are not chemically the same as benzodiazepines but they sedate as the tranquillisers and barbiturates did and should therefore have been viewed with scepticism. Again, in the constant replay of drug history, they were marketed as relatively side-effect free and non-addictive and were therefore believed to be so. But they do produce dependence—something recognised by NICE, and they do lead to withdrawal symptoms. As benzodiazepine prescriptions have fallen, Z drug prescriptions have risen.

Along with Z drugs came the SSRIs. Just as Hoffmann-La Roche formulated a deliberate tactic to oust barbiturates with the benzodiazepine tranquillisers—Valium and Librium, now the manufacturers of the new antidepressants formulated plans to displace benzodiazepines from the market. Drug companies sponsored international symposia attended by hundreds and sometimes thousands of doctors where the harm benzodiazepines were doing was exploited and the efficacy for anxiety of SSRIs acting on serotonin was stressed.

And once again the needle has stuck in the same groove—patients have discovered through personal experience (just as they had previously with benzodiazepines and Z drugs), that the SSRIs were not as harmlessly beneficial as they had been billed. SSRIs, like benzodiazepines, produced a withdrawal reaction when they were stopped. And just as they had accepted without question the message on tranquillisers and hypnotics, doctors and regulators accepted the drug company message that SSRIs were non-addictive. Just as in times past, manufacturers, regulators and the medical profession are fighting to the last (until something new comes along) against a bulwark of Department of Health denial.

Doctors and regulators should have known that since benzodiazepines could replace barbiturates, they were therefore likely to prove addictive. The same people should have known that SSRIs would be likely to be so, since the older tricyclic and MAOI antidepressants had been shown in the early 1980s to produce withdrawal effects. But as always, the faith of regulators and doctors trumped science and they accepted what the manufacturers told them:

> "It seems that Big Pharma is slowly strangling the medical profession, like ivy growing up a tree, and forcing medical complicity with drug company aims, resulting in new definitions of dependence and even new classes of mental illness. How has the industry obtained this insidious stranglehold on the profession? It seems clear that money, not science, is driving pharmacology. Yet the drug companies are the only ones with the funds to conduct large drug trials and to develop new drugs which can, and have, saved many lives; and doctors persist in the belief that a drug will be found that is the answer to each mental illness. There appear to be failures in the whole system under which we have insidiously come to operate."
> Professor Heather Ashton

For a drug company, a favourable trial review is worth whole forests of advertising pages, which is why manufacturers will sometimes spend half a million pounds or more on reprints for worldwide distribution. Unlike advertising, favourable coverage of a drug trial in an influential medical journal confers the medical seal of science approval.

> "Journals have devolved into information laundering operations for the pharmaceutical industry."
> Richard Horton (Editor of the Lancet), Public Library of Science Medical Journal, May 17 2005

When Merck's Vioxx became a blockbuster drug, it has been said that an article in the New England Journal of Medicine which failed to report the dangers, had a lot to do with it. As the LA Times reported, the article cited only selective data on heart attacks and strokes, which allowed Merck to claim that Vioxx was safe for patients with no history of these problems. In December 2005, the Wall Street Journal reported on a 1999 document that came to light in litigation. The document described Pfizer's strategy for publishing articles in medical journals to market its antidepressant Zoloft. It had been prepared by an advertising agency—WPP. It had listed 81 different proposed articles for journals to "promote the drug's use in conditions from panic disorder to paedophilia."

The methodology used in trials and reported in journals, often gives a distorted picture because the research is carried out in a way that ensures that a positive result will be demonstrated. One favourite technique is to remove all subjects who might respond favourably to a placebo before a study begins. For several weeks, prospective trial subjects are given a placebo and observed in what is referred to as the placebo "wash-out" period. Those subjects who improve on a placebo are washed out. This is one way in which, when the study proper begins, the drug is shown to be more effective than placebo. Even then, the 'proved' benefit may be marginal as Professor David Healy and others have found when analysing SSRI data:

> "It is doubtful, that the two-point average advantage for the drugs is meaningful in the real world in which patients function every day, or that the drugs would have had even that slight advantage over placebo had it not been for the wash-out methodology."
> Joseph Wyatt and Donna Midkiff, Biological Psychiatry, 2006

The authors of an article in the BMJ in January 2007, (Harlan Krumholz, Harold Hines, Joseph S. Ross, Amos H. Presler, David S. Egilman), showed how the major medical journals are to blame for their role in transmitting scientifically inaccurate reports which are then widely broadcast to physicians and trotted out without question in public pronouncements. The article examined Vioxx and the evidence showing that even as Merck's own chief scientist, Dr. Edward Scolnick was expressing concerns about the cardiovascular risks, the company submitted a slanted version of the VIGOR report—which was then published in The New England Journal of Medicine.

> "The journals published the studies, and the academic community accepted the findings without expressing much concern."

The authors pointed out that although Merck and the NEJM eventually admitted that the published VIGOR analysis was wrong, none of the academic authors who backed it (all paid by Merck) accepted responsibility or admitted error.

Another favoured technique in trials of psychotropic drugs is to ensure that participants in studies are taken off all medication shortly before the trial begins. Half of the patients are given the trialled drug and half are given a placebo. These studies make a new drug look effective because no one draws attention to the fact that patients in the placebo group may be going through withdrawal from an existing addictive medication.

In a humorous (but only on the surface) article in the BMJ entitled 'Harlot plc' (an amalgamation of the world's two oldest professions), David L. Sackett and Andrew D. Oxman explored how drug companies produce the results they want. These are the most pertinent ones:

- Cite only those reports that support your product, proposal, or policy (and which denigrate your competitor's)
- Give insufficient doses of your competitor's product, accompanied by serious warnings about its side-effects and toxicity
- Scan repeated early analyses for spurious but favourable trends that justify terminating the trial in your favour
- Over-interpret a positive or an indeterminate trial
- Provide generous research grants, first class travel, luxurious accommodations, exorbitant honorariums, and gargantuan ongoing "consultant" fees to "experts" who (surprise) favour your product, screening test, or programme
- Hire celebrities who will promote your 'disease' and tout your product or screening test
- Give generous "journalism" awards for articles that sell your disease or praise your product in the lay media
- Secretly fund patients' action groups to attack any counter evidence that shows your product, programme, or screening test is useless or harmful
- Threaten to move your product development and manufacture to another country

That drug company research and development often serves marketing strategies more than sound science and patient safety has been demonstrated beyond doubt. The medical journals have realised it but the drug regulators, government and many doctors it appears, have not. The majority of media articles continually demonstrate the pre-eminence of its adopted and comfortable role as 'repeater and stenographer', churning out an unquestioning view of new drugs. The following list, shorter than that cited by Harlot comes from various medical journals including JAMA, the New England Journal of Medicine, the British Medical Journal and Lancet:

- Multiple studies are undertaken, and the most favourable ones are chosen for licence applications and the rest are suppressed
- Drug effectiveness is measured in multiple ways and only the best measures are published. The studies chosen for publishing may have little to do with whether patients will be helped
- Professional writers are hired to prepare articles according to company guidelines using favourable phrases and terms selected by the drug companies
- High profile experts are hired to put their names to drug-company-generated articles, although the experts have not participated in the studies and their financial connections with the drug companies are not disclosed

In a BMJ article in 2003 entitled, 'No More Free Lunches' BMJ.2003; 326: 181–1222, the deputy editor Kamran Abbasi, and the editor Richard Smith wrote:

> "Drug development and marketing is a multi-billion dollar industry, where financial interests influence the design and planning of clinical trials. Many tricks can be used to give companies the results they want, including comparing the new drug with a placebo rather than a standard, evidence based treatment or comparing the new drug with an inappropriate existing drug or with too low a dose of the existing drug. Two new studies support these concerns. A systematic review by North American researchers finds that studies sponsored by pharmaceutical companies are four times as likely to have outcomes favouring the sponsor than are studies funded by other independent sources. European researchers look at placebo-controlled studies of the SSRIs and find a literature riddled with multiple and selective publication of studies showing significant drug effects..."

The stakes are enormous and the tactics to keep the money rolling in after a drug is licensed are many and varied. The pharmaceutical group Eli Lilly made £1.8bn from Prozac in 2000 and, seeing the end of its patent, began the now familiar drug company tactic of trying to register the drug for new uses, thereby extending the period of profit. In 2001 it succeeded in getting its life renewed as Sarafem, for severe premenstrual tension, which ensured continuing profit until 2007.

Astra Zeneca produced Nexium (for heartburn) in 2001, just as the existing drug Prilosec was coming to the end of its patent. Nexium was the same drug as Prilosec except for a missing and perhaps non-acting form of the omeprazole molecule. Sure enough Nexium went on to replace the older drug in the financial charts.

Research funding is a primary weapon backing Pharma control of profit margins and science. Merck, the makers of Vioxx and Gardasil, controlled all aspects of the 2002 study reported in the Annals of Internal Medicine, extolling the virtues of Fosamax for osteoporosis. Merck recruited and paid for the 300+ patients involved; collected the data from the trials facilities, and controlled the design and execution of the trials. Merck also retained full control and ownership of the research itself. But media coverage of the research conducted by Dr Susan Greenspan, failed to explore this reality. Fosamax made a great deal of money by targeting young women using the prevention message. With echoes of the current Gardasil campaign which is to 'prevent' the HPV virus causing cervical cancer by vaccinating all young girls (and hopefully boys), Fosamax was marketed extensively and successfully for young women on the premise that taking the drug daily early in life would prevent osteoporosis. Fosamax has now been linked to jaw bone death which involves severe pain and disfigurement. In July 2006, the LA Times said:

> "As Merck & Co. defends itself against a deluge of litigation involving its pain reliever Vioxx, the pharmaceutical giant also is fielding the first of what could be another wave of lawsuits involving Fosamax, its second-biggest seller."

This scenario of funding influence, research control and advertising blitz, producing a licensed drug which is rapidly and widely prescribed, before patients then discover the harm, happens time and time again.

On September 21, 2006, an FDA Advisory Committee met to review negative research findings on Bayer's Trasylol, which is used to control bleeding in open heart surgery. The panel initially decided that there was no need for any additional warning on Trasylol. But, in giving its evidence, somehow Bayer "forgot to mention" the findings of a study of 67,000 patients which it had commissioned itself that confirmed the risks associated with Trasylol. Bayer had received the results seven days before the examination. It was one of the researchers who had been involved in the study who enlightened the FDA. The FDA then issued an advisory note saying the results of the study demonstrate:

> "...that use of Trasylol may increase the chance for death, serious kidney damage, congestive heart failure and strokes."

Then there is the disingenuity of GSK with its antidepressant Seroxat:

> "Panorama's account [BBC programme] of GlaxoSmithKline's successful attempts to market Seroxat for use in children, despite the fact that its own published trial found evidence of serious adverse effects and failed to show benefit, is fascinating but depressingly familiar. What is even more depressing is that such behaviour is still so widely tolerated within medicine." Legislation is not going to happen soon—the powerful industry lobby will make sure of that. Regulation is still inadequate. So what can we do to change the blind-eye culture of medicine? In the interests of patients and professional integrity I suggest intolerance and exposure."
> BMJ Editor, Fiona Godlee, 29 January 2007

Dr David Healy has calculated that a quarter of a million people worldwide have tried to commit suicide because of Prozac and that 25,000 have succeeded. Healy has said that in a past conversation he had with Professor Charles Nemeroff, he told him that it was their duty as doctors to warn of the side-effects of drugs, to make them as safe as possible. Nemeroff, Chairman of the Department of Psychiatry and Behavioural sciences at Emory University replied that it was immaterial what people like him or Healy did. Drug companies were answerable to their shareholders and profit was the bottom line.

In September 2004, in a joint editorial, eleven medical journals including the British Medical Journal told researchers and firms to register trials at the start so negative or unclear results could not be covered up. The medical journals said that they would no longer publish articles about study results unless producers publicly registered the tests on Web sites like ClinicalTrials.gov, which is run by the National Library of Medicine.

As part of the settlement between GlaxoSmithKline and New York Attorney General Eliot Spitzer, GSK agreed to release information on all its clinical studies. The first information posted on a new website by GSK related to 65 studies involving its diabetes drug, Avandia. Dr. Steven Nissen, a cardiologist at the Cleveland Clinic, having discovered the GSK website, produced an analysis of the data showing that Avandia led to a greater cardiac risk. GSK is of course denying this.

On 1 October 2004, a registry of trials data was launched on the internet by the Pharmaceutical Research and Manufacturers of America containing summaries of findings since 2002. However, a deputy editor of JAMA, Dr

Drummond Rennie said that while it was progress, his experience of drug companies led him to believe that it was:

> "...unlikely that [the] industry will ever be able to establish a large, common, complete, useful, trustworthy, up-to-date and easily accessible register."

David Healy said in January 2005 that the trials information so far revealed by GSK and Eli Lilly had not been ideal:

> "They don't put all the raw data and things that can be of the greatest interest [on the web]...You still get a spin on the data that's more favourable to the company."

In October 2006 it was reported that Cancer United, a European umbrella campaign, was to push for equality of cancer care across the European Union. As it turned out the campaign was being entirely funded by Roche, the maker of cancer drugs Herceptin and Avastin. A Roche executive had a place on the board and the Roche Public Relations company was providing the secretariat. The main study on which the campaign was based, which is controversial, was funded by Roche. The goal was obvious—to press governments to fund increases in expenditure on the Roche drugs, backed up by Roche produced science with claims that patient survival is linked to the amount that government spends on drugs. Dr Michel Coleman from the London School of Hygiene and Tropical Medicine said:

> "Cancer patient groups should think twice before accepting sponsorship from Cancer United."

In 2006 in the journal Public Library of Science Medicine, experts from across the world argued that new diseases are being defined by those who are often linked to the pharmaceutical industry. They argued that sales are being increased through the medicalisation of normal life:

> "It is in the interests of pharmaceutical companies to extend the range of the abnormal so that the market for treatments is proportionately enlarged."
> Dr Iona Heath, London GP, 2005

Ray Moynihan and David Henry wrote in the editorial:

> "Informal alliances of pharmaceutical corporations, public relations firms, doctors' groups and patient advocates promote

these ideas to the public and policy makers, often using mass media to push a certain view of a particular health problem."

The aspects of normal life, activity and emotion being promoted by drug companies as illnesses needing drug treatment include:

Erectile dysfunction: A particular concern of Pfizer which says that 50% of men over forty have difficulties achieving or maintaining an erection.
Female sexual dysfunction: This condition has no real definition and has been described as preconceived with no evidence base. In the BMJ in 2005, Dr Leonore Tiefer, a clinical professor of psychiatry at New York University, said on the subject of the Proctor and Gamble campaign for the licensing of testosterone patches for women, "The product the company is selling at this stage is really the disease. I think Proctor and Gamble has a marketing plan that worked for shampoo. Create a buzz, get the word out, heighten consciousness—get people talking."
ADHD: The particular concern of Eli Lilly and Co, Novartis AG, Johnson & Johnson, and Shire plc. Prescriptions for ADHD drugs have rocketed since the 1990s following Pharma sponsored involvement of educationalists in diagnosis and dissemination of information to parents. Take a look at the web, it is plastered with pro articles and advertising.
Bipolar disorder: In one of the eleven PLOS papers, Professor David Healy described how a TV advertisement from Eli Lilly encouraged people to find out about mood disorders through a website sponsored by the company. He described bipolar disorder as "the latest mania."
Restless legs syndrome: This it seems is seen as a widespread condition by GlaxoSmithKline which launched its awareness campaign in 2003 and fortuitously only two years later had the drug Ropinirole, to treat the condition.
Shopping Addiction: The antidepressant drug citalopram is highly regarded in some quarters as a treatment for the addiction.
Road Rage: Two antidepressants, fluoxetine and divalproex are being trialled in the US. As researchers say, "It is a vaguely defined condition for which effective treatments have not been identified. "

It might be interesting to examine which of these aspects could possibly be part of your own life or the lives of those you know. You might then compile a definitive list of the drugs you and they need and should be taking.

The closet financial relationships between drug manufacturers and psychiatry's leading "experts" who decide what constitutes a "mental disorder" were clearly described in April 2006 by Lisa Cosgrove and Sheldon Krimsky. The DSM is psychiatry's diagnostic holy book published by the American Psychiatric Association. One hundred percent of the members of the panels on Mood Disorders and Schizophrenia and other Psychotic Disorders it appears had financial ties to drug companies. These are the most profitable categories of mental illness because this is the area where most drugs are prescribed. In 2004 antidepressants had total world sales of $20.3 billion. Antipsychotics had total annual sales of $14.1 billion —and these figures are rising rapidly. The study found that most of the money received by the DSM-IV panellists was for their research. The DSM is carefully constructed and according to David Healy, if a condition does not respond to 'preferred' drugs, the condition is dropped from the bible. Preferred drugs are of course usually the ones which are associated with the rising influential careers of the panellists. As Dr. Irwin Savodnik, an assistant clinical professor of psychiatry at the University of California said:

> "The very vocabulary of psychiatry is now defined at all levels by the pharmaceutical industry."

In December 2006, using a decade of secret documents, the New York Times described how Eli Lilly had kept information from doctors about Zyprexa's links to obesity and its tendency to raise blood sugar—both known risk factors for diabetes. Instead of warning doctors and patients, Lilly told its sales representatives to play the dangers down, being more concerned that Zyprexa's sales would be hurt if the company told the truth about the fact that the drug might cause unmanageable weight gain or diabetes. In 2002 Lilly rejected plans to give psychiatrists guidance about how to treat diabetes, worrying that to do so would tarnish Zyprexa's reputation. Instead it increased its marketing to GPs. In February 2007, FDA scientist Dr David Graham, who exposed Merck and Vioxx, testified at a US House of Representatives Energy and Commerce sub-committee hearing and said the off-label use of antipsychotics like Zyprexa to sedate nursing home residents kills roughly 15,000 people a year. Dr Graham also told members of the committee that Lilly and the FDA had known for a long time that Zyprexa caused weight gain that could lead to diabetes.

> "With Vioxx, Merck and the F.D.A. acted out of ruthless, short-sighted, and irresponsible self-interest."
> Richard Horton, Editor of the Lancet

In May 2003, the Guardian reported the former editor of the BMJ, Richard Smith saying that fraudulent research regularly appears in the 30,000 scientific journals published worldwide. He said:

> "Most cases are not publicised. They are simply not recognised, covered up altogether, or the guilty researcher is

> urged to retrain, move to another institution or retire from research."

Patients are of course on the end of that research.

In May 2007 the Independent reported on a first-of-its-kind legal quest by Pfizer and marketing partner Eisai of Japan to have a decision of the National Institute for Health and Clinical Excellence overturned. The judicial review of the NICE guidance on Alzheimer's drugs came at the end of a two-year battle over access to Eisai and Pfizer's Aricept, Shire's Reminyl, and Novartis' Exelon for sufferers of the disease. It is perhaps the first sign of a growing gap between the pharmaceutical industry and government. The UK government set up NICE to vet drugs for value and NICE came up with a rejection of the Alzheimer drugs. The worry for drug companies is that the NICE approach could be exported to other countries. In 2006, Pfizer was not best pleased when NICE gave only limited approval for Exubera, the first inhaled insulin system for diabetics.

The patient group the Alzheimer's Society has led a populist campaign against the NICE ruling that the dementia drugs should not be provided by the NHS. Figures from the charities show that in the financial year before the judicial review was sought, the Alzheimer's Society received £31,000 from Pfizer and Eisai, which makes Aricept. The society also received £13,000 from Shire Pharmaceuticals, manufacturer of Reminyl, and £14,000 from Novartis, manufacturer of Exelon.

Big Pharma continually lobbies ministers about NICE decisions. After they had solicited the influence of the White House for their cause, the US deputy health secretary, Alex Azar, had meaningful conversations with the UK health secretary, Patricia Hewitt in 2006, where he explained his belief that a free market for the largely US-based major drug companies was a good direction to go in. The White House lobbying is part of the strategy of the US pharma-political complex to allow the world's main drug companies unrestricted access to the NHS. They describe it as free market reform.

Azar used the drug company argument that any form of control (in this case NICE control) would impact on innovation. Looking into his crystal ball he said that if all new drugs were automatically approved, companies would fight it out and this would result in cheaper drugs. Alex Azar now works for a major pharmaceutical company:

Azar says that an unrestricted flow of drugs will keep people out of hospital, thereby cutting NHS costs. On that score, it is known that drug side-effects cause the deaths of thousands of patients who end up in hospital each year. In 2006 the British Medical Association said that at least 250,000 people are admitted to hospital every year because of the damaging side-effects of the medicines they are taking. But for a politician or a drug company executive—facts like that should never be allowed to interfere with established procedure and profit.

> "[There is] a social contract involving drug producers, drug prescribers, drug regulators, and information suppliers. In a properly functioning society, openness and honesty should be assumed and certain standards of behaviour expected. Indeed, in an ideal world, drug companies should be trusted."
> Joe Collier, Professor of Medicines Policy and Consultant in Clinical Pharmacology, St George's Hospital and Medical School, London, BMJ.2007; 334: 209 January 27 2007

The drug company and BMA argument is that medicine is now so closely scrutinised and regulated, with prescribing largely dictated by evidence-based guidance, that it is far harder for doctors to be influenced into inappropriate prescribing. The secondary argument is that doctors are professionals whose judgement is above influence. It is true that the days of excessive hospitality are ostensibly over, since the Association of the British Pharmaceutical Industry (ABPI) brought in a new code of conduct on 1 January 2006. Under it, promotion to doctors should cost no more than £6 plus VAT. The gift has to be relevant to professional practice and travel expenses cannot be paid for attending local meetings. All flights are economy only (unless you are a speaker).

A poll of GPs in July 2007 conducted by consumer group 'Which?' found that doctors received four visits per month on average from drug reps. One GP had twenty-two companies contacting her about thirty-one drugs in one month. Doctors received five promotional mailings about new drugs a week, and there were also invitations to attend conferences. A quarter of the GPs questioned had been sponsored to attend a conference, seminar or training event in the UK in the previous twelve months and 5% had been sponsored to attend an event abroad. But Pharma sees nothing wrong with this:

> "I make no apologies for the fact that pharmaceutical companies are in close contact with doctors about new medicines. It is right and proper that they inform GPs about new medicines, and how they might benefit their patients, so that doctors are kept up to date."
> Richard Ley, ABPI

There is abundant evidence that advertising works. The more heavily advertised a drug, the greater the sales, and the greater the number of prescriptions, compared to similar but less advertised drugs. More worryingly, the apparent incidence of the illnesses at which the drugs are aimed also increases. According to David Healy, the effective incidence of depression, OCD, social phobia and PTSD has increased one thousand-fold worldwide since 1980.

> "Strong reasons exist for **not** seeing representatives. Their job is primarily to sell their company's product. They are an important part of the pharmaceutical industry's promotion methods, and they are highly successful in altering doctors' prescribing habits. Not surprisingly, there is also evidence that the more reliant [that] doctors are on commercial sources of information, the less rational they are as prescribers."
> David Griffith, Consultant Physician for Care of Older People, Mayday Healthcare, Surrey

The drug manufacturers spend £1.65bn marketing their drugs annually in the UK. On the other hand the Department of Health has been spending a mere £4.5m a year providing independent prescribing information to doctors. That figure reduced in 2006, when it eliminated its financing for the independent Drugs and Therapeutics Bulletin (DTB).

Researchers and physicians who write the rules on prescribing drugs have extensive financial connections with the pharmaceutical industry, an investigation by the journal Nature revealed in October 2005. Nature found that more than one-third of authors declared financial links to relevant drug companies, with around 70% of panels being affected. In one case, every member of the panel had been paid by the company responsible for the drug that was ultimately recommended. Drummond Rennie, deputy editor of the Journal of the American Medical Association said:

> "Drug company sponsors see guideline-issuing bodies as perfect places to exert influence. The practice stinks."

As Marcia Angell pointed out in 'The Truth About the Drug Companies', the great majority of innovative 'new' drugs are not innovative at all but merely variations of existing drugs. 'Me-toos are an easy route to profit. Moreover, even innovative drugs are often not produced by Pharma itself, but are licensed from universities or biotech companies. The FDA approved seventy-eight drugs in 2002 and only seventeen contained new active ingredients, and a mere seven of these were seen as improvements over older drugs. Instead of researching new cures, companies manipulate older drugs to gain a new patent. Then they conduct trials which are intended to find anything that they can market as something new in their advertising.

The biggest single item in a drug company budget is not Research and Development but something vaguely named Marketing and Administration.

As the pipeline of new drugs shrinks, marketing and administration expands and becomes more and more a Pharma priority.

Contemporary pharmaceutical marketing practices are a continuation of 19th Century quack medicine advertising. Potion sellers invented 'medical' advertising and strategies to create demand. Pharmaceutical marketing is more closely allied to advertising for soap powder and makeup than it is to medicine. The pharmaceutical companies have based their strategies on the idea of never-ending personal needs, which in their own specialist sphere they seek to provide, as a means to profit. Campaigns targeting and using the strategy of prevention, improvement and life-enhancement have created stratospheric profits through new 'essential' drugs—such as anti-psychotics, SSRIs, hypnotics, drugs for allergies, cholesterol reduction, insomnia, and heartburn. The messages say these are vital for daily and lifelong physical and mental well-being.

For Pharma, patients are not patients at all, but consumers, as doctors became long since. Promoting consumer familiarity with drugs is a strategy used successfully in New Zealand and in the US. Pharma has already incorporated medical journals, drug regulators, doctors, politicians, the media, the law, patients groups, ethics committees and academia into its mission statement. Through direct advertising it seeks to incorporate the final and most vital frontier—patients.

The pharmaceutical industry finds it easy to link ethical objectives to its marketing activities. Who can argue against a company which says that what is done is being done in the attempt to alleviate suffering? Gardasil is taking the medical world by storm in the name of protecting women from sexually transmitted disease, but it should be remembered that Gardasil is made by Merck who also made the painkiller Vioxx. Pharma always maintains the view that directly influencing patients/consumers is beneficial to their needs and leads to empowerment. All this is an illusion and a smokescreen. Maryland psychiatrist Jack E. Rosenblatt, editor of 'Currents in Affective Illness' says:

> "Drug makers don't seem to realize that this is not toothpaste or shampoo—that they are dealing with something that can really hurt people."

In spite of the large numbers of doubtful trials, manufacturers seldom see the necessity of conducting post marketing studies to ensure new drugs are really safe.

> "There is no incentive for companies to find problems with safety once a drug is approved. It is just downside risk. We find out a drug is unsafe when the bodies accumulate."
> Denis Mangano, Ischemia Research & Education Foundation, California.

> "The whole process [trials] has been corrupted. It is getting worse as the financial stakes are rising."
> Dr Aubrey Blumsohn, former lead researcher on Actonel for Procter and Gamble

In November 2004, The Observer examined how in 1998, GSK, the UK's biggest drug company, had drawn up a plan to double sales of the SSRI Seroxat/Paxil through marketing it as a cure for a range of other conditions. This was in spite of much patient evidence that the drug was linked with suicide and a number of very serious withdrawal symptoms. The 1999 internal document outlined how GSK intended to market Seroxat for social anxiety disorder. Professor David Healy said:

> "What this document makes clear is that a number of different forms of anxiety were being targeted in a systematic way. The thrust was to move sales beyond the $1 billion to the $2 billion mark by pushing it to people who were not clinically depressed."

> "It is [for example] becoming increasing apparent that scientific findings relating to the risk of suicide with some commonly used antidepressants have been distorted. University academics were [again] involved in fronting misleading science. Incomplete information was provided by companies to authoring academics and the regulators, and this information was simply accepted with blind faith."
> Dr Aubrey Blumsohn

In 1999, the media discovered the case of Boots Pharmaceuticals and Betty Dong who was a researcher at the University of California in San Francisco. In 1990 she was researching the Boots thyroid drug Synthroid. She found through the research that Synthroid had serious side-effects. In what has become a time-honoured Pharma approach to unpalatable research discoveries, she was threatened with legal action if she published her findings. It was only after the media became involved that her findings were disclosed. In 1999/2000 Boots paid $170 million to settle lawsuits. But it has been estimated that the company made a profit of $3billion during these years. This is what owning the research means for drug companies, they are able to control unwelcome findings which would hit profits. By the time the facts come into the open, the profits have been made, shareholders have benefited and the harm done to patients becomes a minor debit on the balance sheet.

Other high profile cases involved Dr. David Healy and Nancy Olivieri. Healy lost an academic position at the University of Toronto in 2000 after he made his views known regarding Prozac and suicide in patients. At the time, the university had received a $1.5 million gift from Eli Lilly, the manufacturer of Prozac. Olivieri, a researcher in paediatric haematology at the same university was also threatened with legal action by Apotex who did not like what was being said about its product deferiprone which she was researching. She lost her job at the university and it later emerged that the University had been seeking grants from Apotex of $55 million.

Another academic who found his university less than helpful when he revealed Pharma misconduct was Dr Aubrey Blumsohn, a researcher at Sheffield in the UK. Dr. Blumsohn had attempted, in vain, to get access to the data from a research project that he was ostensibly leading, and to control the writing of research abstracts. His attempts, as is the norm, were opposed by the drug company involved—Procter & Gamble. Sheffield University failed to support Blumsohn, and suspended him after he talked to the media about the situation. Dr Blumsohn and the University later parted company, the doctor receiving an undisclosed settlement. As he wrote later:

> "With governments setting the standard for scientific conduct, it is hardly surprising that industry-recruited academic "thought leaders" (perhaps academic prostitutes) continue to function with impunity."

In 1997 with Prozac, and years later with Seroxat, David Healy had gained access to undisclosed data in his capacity as an expert witness in a legal action. This is the way that most of what becomes known about the real evidence of efficacy and harm is discovered—through legal actions in the US. It is well nigh impossible to sue a drug company in Britain, mainly due to the difficulties placed in the way of acquiring the necessary funding to pursue an individual or group action, and so discoveries by expert witnesses do not normally occur. But the drugs are the same here as in the US, though maybe with a different name. It is easy to imagine how patients in the UK feel when they see legal cases proceeding in the US when they took the same drug but have no access to the law.

Hidden evidence on other drugs has emerged over the years through US legal actions such as Vioxx and Zyprexa but the UK system of medicine regulation is such that no one answers for having knowingly hidden dangers and exposing patients to preventable harm for profit. No one takes responsibility and no one is forced to take responsibility.

A BBC Panorama programme on 29 January 2007 showed how GSK, the company making Seroxat distorted evidence that the drug raised the risk of suicide in children. The secret documents showed how GSK had distorted what was once the gold standard system for analysing drug safety and effectiveness—the clinical trial. Until relatively recently, trials were overwhelmingly conducted in universities, independently of drug companies but increasingly these are now conducted and controlled by the drug companies themselves. Now company employees oversee the data.

Neither regulators nor governments and certainly not the law control the 'health' corporations' injury carousel. No new revelation of deliberate falsification brings with it any consequences, beyond what US law extracts. In the UK there are no consequences, financial or otherwise. The mantra from Big Pharma is always the same, they acted in good time when they became aware, and all drugs have some side-effects. All drugs do have side-effects, but they are frequently side-effects which are hidden and which then kill and maim patients unnecessarily. But the drug companies still thrive, and each new drug—even from a company with a history, is welcomed with open arms by regulators and the medical profession.

> "We've created an impression with the American public that when a drug is approved, it's perfectly safe. We have not done a good job about educating the patients of America that all drugs come with significant side-effects."
> Billy Tauzin, President of the Pharmaceutical Research and Manufacturers of America, lobbyists for the drug industry.

Billy Tauzin, prior to his current very lucrative position as head of PhRMA, was heading a congressional investigation into drug company practices. The damaging practices still continue.

The UK Drugs regulator, the MHRA has never taken any action against academics making fraudulent claims in ghost written articles, or doctors working for the companies who repeat such claims. Aubrey Blumsohn has had this to say:

> "The MHRA says it has no legal remit to investigate scientific fraud in pharmaceutical research after it has licensed a drug —that it has no remit to investigate ghost writing by companies on behalf of university academics. The MHRA have also stated that they have no procedure for investigation of scientific fraud. Finally it claims that the fact that a scientist

obtained some raw data pertaining to information written in his name without the consent of a company is "illegal"!"

In February 2007, Charles Medawar gave a reminder that the regulator had (so it said) begun an investigation into GSK and Seroxat in October 2003. The investigation may still not be going on in July 2007. As he wrote:

> "The reality is that any prosecution of the Company would put the Agency itself—and Chairman Breckenridge in particular—too squarely in the frame. What was it he told Panorama for the second of their four splendid programmes (11May 2003)—"What you can say with great firmness is that these drugs do not increase the risk of suicidal thought and they do not increase the risk of suicide.""

With the departure of T. Blair and the arrival in 10, Downing Street of one G. Brown, another good reason for not doing anything about Seroxat may have emerged. A new Business Council is to be set up and its functions are described as to "look at, adjudicate upon and inquire into the [business] policies we are pursuing." Among the luminary membership is one Jean-Paul Garnier—he is of course the CEO of GlaxoSmithKline, the makers of Seroxat.

The only other body to turn to is the General Medical Council, whose job it is to investigate the conduct of doctors—but it has shown no inclination to protect. On several occasions, benzodiazepine campaigners have asked the GMC to act on the over-prescription issue, but sadly there has never been a reply.

The main contributory factor in the ongoing slide of drug medicine into medical assault, and one which cannot be over-emphasised is that in the UK, the Department of Health looks after both the drug industry and public health. While that situation continues, the health of the patient will always take second place to the health of the industry. Patients' welfare will always remain as a footnote while government health policies and practice are dominated by the influence of unaccountable corporations.

No life is sacred to Pharma, from that of a child to that of the oldest member of society. Drug companies worship only the balance sheet. That way their shareholder responsibilities are fulfilled and shareholders are the only controllers they recognise.

Conclusion

Pharmageddon:

"The prospect of a world in which medicines and medicine produce more ill-health than health, and when medical progress does more harm than good"

Definition formulated at a Seminar in London in April 2007

Heresy historically meant holding a religious belief which the Church disagreed with; treason meant trying to overthrow the government (sometimes by thought). Today in medicine, heresy is a belief in something other than the message which comes ultimately from the pharmaceutical companies. Holding divergent beliefs is seen by the establishment providers of medicine as something akin to treason—an attempt to overthrow the comfortable and public declarations of its interdependent insider view. In George Orwell's dystopian novel 'Nineteen Eighty-Four', the government attempted to control individual beliefs, labelling disapproved of thoughts with the term "crimethink". The first Elizabethan Age was an age when Sir Francis Walsingham decreed that certain intellectual efforts were crimes punishable by death. For insiders in medicine today, uttering challenging, non-approved views on medicine, its benefits and its dangers, is no longer punishable by death. Instead it leads to the lesser punishments of ostracism, isolation, scorn and ridicule. For patients as the receivers however, death sentences may be involved, since the result of the cosy and incestuous philosophies held by providers is often the denial of truth about the potential for injury.

The tranquilliser story is not the story of an accident; of something unfortunate happening to a few while the majority were cured of a threatening illness. The risk/benefit equation would seem at best to have been based on an establishment view of there being acceptable numbers of casualties of a largely beneficial and needed drug—an insignificant detail compared with the numbers saved from a serious condition. I say at best, because even today, most of what the drugs cause is actively denied, downplayed and disregarded. And tranquillisers were never in the main life-saving drugs which it was worthwhile to take a risk on—they were largely sticking plasters for consciousness. The problem has been that for huge numbers of people the sticking plaster turned out to be non-sterile and a carrier of infection. The story has been one where few who were over prescribed remained unaffected in some degree. Patients could and should have been protected by a drugs regulatory system which cared more for patients and much less for its own indoctrinated belief in drugs and false beliefs in its own expertise. Aubrey Blumsohn said in July 2007:

> "The system seems to operate as if the truth is optional. I have no doubt that regulatory malfunction is behind many of our troubles in medicine. The MHRA is a disreputable organisation that has on occasion enabled the mingling of disinformation with distortion and plain lies..."

Patients could and should have been protected by the politicians who received heartfelt experiences by the shed-load, the victims having found that medicine remained aloof from the injury it had caused. But the politicians, when they did comment, paid lip service to what they termed 'the problem' and by and large allowed the situation to continue. What happens to politicians once they achieve power and responsibility—divorcing them from the human roots they sprang from and the feelings they presumably once had? Why is it that politics seems to value the denial of fact more than protection of the innocent?

The Pharmaceutical companies which inflicted such injury through tranquillisers—life improvement drugs, have now moved big time into the Protection Racket—the marketing of preventative medicines. Vaccinations are seen as the money-spinners of the future. And how could anyone be opposed to protecting children or preventing the HPV virus? Government and medicine have quickly answered that question for themselves as—no one. They are determined to repeat the mistakes of the past and give a turbo-boost to the enterprise. The Government's defence of the MMR vaccine—that no clear link has been proven between the MMR and autism—are extremely misleading. When evidence emerged that there could be a problem, as usual they rejected or ignored it. Dr Peter Fletcher, a former Government drugs safety officer said in 2006 that he had seen a "steady accumulation of evidence" from scientists worldwide that the measles, mumps and rubella jab is causing brain damage in certain children. He has referred to the:

> "...very powerful people who have staked their reputations and careers on the safety of MMR and are willing to do almost anything to protect themselves."

UK children can receive 25 vaccines by the age of 15 months—many of which are for illnesses with little risk today. Cervical cancer is not what anyone would want any woman to experience, but it is not at all common. In the UK it forms just below 1.5 per cent of cancer deaths. Merck's Gardasil vaccine only protects against the two types of HPV that cause 70 per cent of this cancer. There is no protection against other strains. Trial subjects were followed up for only two years and therefore there is no knowing how it will affect girls and women in the long-term. Experiences from the past certainly suggest there might be problems. By the 1970s the oral polio vaccine caused more people to become paralysed than polio did. In the UK, between 1968 and 2005, there were 114 reports linking serious encephalitis in children with the measles vaccine though by the 1950s there were fewer than 100 deaths per year from measles. For most of the 20th Century the death rate from mumps has remained at about ten or twenty a year. Vaccines have raised the age at which mumps is caught from early childhood—when the illness is usually mild—into adolescence when it is much more likely to be severe. Medicine has paid so little attention to the damage it may cause—despite the historical instruction "first, do no harm."

At the end of June 2007, the National Institute for Clinical Excellence issued new guidelines on statins, which according to them should be prescribed to people with a 20% risk of developing heart disease. Statins include Crestor, Lipitor and Zocor The marketing of statins as a protection against heart disease has been intense and long-lasting—the budget for one year for Crestor alone was $1 billion

But do the drugs lead to longer and better quality of life? A report in the Lancet stated that in men who did not already have heart disease, and in all women, there was no evidence that taking statins increased their life by a single day. Figures provided by the Medical Research Council show that if a man took them for thirty years he could possibly live for nine months longer.

The medical establishment has swallowed the Pharma message on these drugs as though it were holy writ but there are a growing number of sceptics, including cardiologists, biochemists and neurologists who say it is possible that statins are a huge waste of money. The cost is enormous, and for the NHS, if testing is included, it could be £5 billion a year—if the NICE guidelines are adopted and followed.

The fear is that regular statin takers are being put at risk of numerous side-effects, some of them potentially fatal. Muscle damage leading to pain and weakness is a common side-effect but some patients develop a severe condition called rhabdomyolysis which can cause kidney failure. In the US there were a total of 416 deaths between 1997 and 2004 solely attributable to Zocor according to the FDA. And it should never be forgotten that reported and attributable deaths due to prescribed drugs are usually the tip of the iceberg in that country and in the UK. Other drug side-effects include cognitive damage, amnesia, anger and impotence. The WHO is now considering the possibility that taking the drugs can lead to amyotrophic lateral dystrophy, a neurological condition which is speedily fatal. As Cheshire GP and cholesterol specialist Dr Malcolm Kendrick says:

> "If you tell your GP of your concern, he or she will most likely dismiss it. But we should be questioning the research and asking hard questions about the role played by the pharmaceutical industry in promoting these drugs."

The Department of Health has no idea how many have been affected by tranquillisers, which is par for the course in medicine, and it does not seem to want to know. But many thousands have told their stories in the media and on the internet. The thousands who died have sadly been unable to tell their stories. Some people who died or who were injured did not themselves take tranquillisers—they were killed or injured in accidents by those who had. The benzodiazepine story is most notable for the number of people it affected because of the huge numbers of people to whom tranquillisers were prescribed. It is a complete description of a medical system which out-sources drug production to private enterprise and then because it has done so, maintains a closed system of regulation which it is almost impossible to penetrate. Establishment medicine and politicians defend what happens to patients in order to defend the system they have jointly created. This is the reason why they show no desire to learn, and continue to learn nothing from the chequered history of drugs.

The tranquilliser story shows clearly what the UK government would not wish included in its description of 'our way of life'. Including what benzodiazepines have done to patients for nearly fifty years might prompt the question, "Is the first duty of the state really the protection of its citizens?" If it is then government has failed to do it. The suspicion has to be that the maintenance of a failing but profitable system is politically more desirable than the introduction of an efficient protective healthcare agenda. The only protections that patients have against drug disasters are the enlightenment of doctors, strictly honest science and effective regulation. All of these health protections have failed in the past, particularly with psychotropic drugs and the true enormity of these failings is illustrated beyond measure by benzodiazepines.

Bibliography

Colin Downes-Grainger 1947 - 2009

Colin's campaigning blogs, pamphlets, letters, satire, cartoons and pictures can be viewed and read on Ray Nimmo's website:

benzo.org.uk

• Camouflage for Medical Practice or Real Assistance? Colin Downes-Grainger, September 11, 2009.

• The Patient is always Right? Colin Downes-Grainger, August 21, 2009.

• Dancing Round the Awful Truth (PDF), Colin Downes-Grainger, July 2, 2009.

• Medical Research on Benzodiazepine Injury (PDF), compiled by Colin Downes-Grainger, June 16, 2009.

• Letter to Department of Health on Protocol (PDF), Colin Downes-Grainger, March 12, 2009.

• The Impossibility of Dialogue with the Department of Health, Colin Downes-Grainger, March 10, 2009.

• Letter to Lord Morris, Colin Downes-Grainger, March 7, 2009.

• Letter to Lord Winston, Colin Downes-Grainger, March 6, 2009.

• A Tale of Two Scandals (PDF), Colin Downes-Grainger, February 25, 2009.

• *Lividicus & the Grim Pill's Progress, Colin Downes-Grainger, February 5, 2009.*

• Illegal v Legal Benzodiazepine addiction, Colin Downes-Grainger, January 28, 2009.

• Letter to Health Minister Dawn Primarolo MP, Colin Downes-Grainger, December 19, 2008.

• Professor David Nutt - a man with a mission (PDF), Colin Downes-Grainger, December 11, 2008.

• Benzo Withdrawal Realities, Colin Downes-Grainger, July 23, 2008.

• State Benefits, Tranquillisers and the DWP, Colin Downes-Grainger, July 22, 2008.

• Tranquilliser Dissonance, Colin Downes-Grainger, July 9, 2008.

• The Lock on Pandora's Box, BBC Watch Politics Show West: Tranquillisers, a Critique, Colin Downes-Grainger, June 24, 2008.

• Tranquilliser Questions - Avoiding Answers (PDF), Colin Downes-Grainger, June 2, 2008.

• Blaming the Patient, (PDF) Colin Downes-Grainger, May 6, 2008.

• Prescription for Injury, Colin Downes-Grainger, August, 2007. Download PDF.

• The First Duty of the State is the Protection of Citizens? (PDF), Colin Downes-Grainger, January 2007.

• An Open Letter on the Human Tragedy of Benzodiazepines in the UK (PDF), Colin Downes-Grainger, January 2006.

• The Story of a 30 Year Addiction to Benzos, Colin Downes-Grainger, September 2002.

Colin's campaigning pictures and cartoons can also be viewed on Emma Holister's website:

www.art-margin.com

His work is in the 'Other Artists' section.

* 9 7 8 1 8 4 4 2 6 8 0 3 0 *

SD - #0034 - 060826 - C0 - 210/148/12 - PB - 9781844268030 - Gloss Lamination